TABLE OF

INTRODUCTION

Alkaline diets are diets that involve eating food that maintains a ph balance above 7. The ph scale is what is used to determine how acidic or alkaline something is. 7 is neutral which means that it is neither acidic or alkaline. Anything above 7 is considered alkaline anything below is considered acidic. Alkaline diets take a list of foods that are considered to be alkaline or that don't create acid in the body when they are digested and recommend that people eat these foods.

Why choose alkaline diets?

Some people believe that the way we eat in today's society is extremely harmful to our health. They believe that eating overly acidic foods is detrimental to the health of the cells and blood of the body. Unfortunately, there has not been many human trials to reference this data scientifically but there have been a number of people who have tried alkaline diets and have reported remarkable health benefits.

Some of the health benefits of Alkaline diets include increased energy, weight loss, less dependence or no dependence on insulin for diabetes patients, no more acid reflux, improved hair, nails, skin, better sleep patterns, mental clarity, relief of symptoms of candida and gout just to name a few. It has also been reported to be very successful in treating cancer. It is true that cancer cells are dormant at a ph of 7.4.

So it makes sense that if you were able to achieve alkalinity within the body that it could improve the condition of cancer, but unfortunately there is not significant scientific data to back up these claims.

1

At the forefront of alkaline diets, is a man by the name of Robert Young. Robert Young is an microbiologist who has been involved with alkalinediets for several decades. He believes alkaline diets to be the cure for all sickness and disease. He has written several books on the subject.

The theory behind alkaline diets is that the body functions naturally in an alkaline state. The blood within your bloodstream, in fact, has a ph of 7.3. Dr. Robert Young states that the body fights tooth and nail to maintain this alkaline balance, but in today's world with our bodies being bombarded by more and more toxins each and every day our bodies are fighting a losing battle causing acid to build up in our systems. This he explains is why diseases such as cancer, arthritis, osteoporosis, etc...

Guildline of alkaline Diet

The alkaline diet is also known as the ph miracle, ph balanced diet, or the acid alkaline diet among other things. It based on the theory that everything that you eat can either cause your body to build up acid or to become more alkaline. For someone starting this diet, it can be overwhelming trying to figure out what is good (alkaline) and what is bad (acidic). This is why I have decided to put together the alkaline diet guidelines and so clear up some of the confusion.

There are many alkaline diet guidelines. The basic idea is certain substances are worse for the body than others. One of the alkaline diet guidelines is that you should attempt to eat 75-80% alkaline. Meaning that 75-80% of your diet is from the alkaline food chart. Certain foods are considered more acid-forming than others though.

To give you an idea here is a list of foods that are considered highly acid forming according to the alkaline diet guidelines:

Sweeteners (equal, sweet and low, neutral-sweet, and aspartame to name a few) beer, table salt, jam, ice cream, beef, lobster, fried food, processed cheese, and soft drinks.Here is a fun fact cola has a ph of 2.5. This is highly acidic. In order to neutralize one can of cola, you would have to drink 32 glasses of water.On the other side of the spectrum, there is a certain food that is considered by highly alkaline and when ingested help increases the alkalinity of the body. According to the alkaline diet guidelines, these food are as follows: sea salt, lotus rood, watermelon, tangerines, sweet potato, lime, pineapple, seaweed, pumpkin seeds, and lentils.

The alkaline diet guidelines say that drugs are extremely acid forming as well. Think about all those people who take some form of the drug to ease their acid reflux. Little do they know their temporary solution is causing bigger problems for them in the long run. There are many other alkaline diet foods this was just an example. The more you eat the better you will feel. Many times people experience a period of detoxification when they switch to the alkaline diet. The alkaline diet guidelines suggest that you got through a period of a couple of weeks in detox to rid your body of toxins and allow to adjust to this completely new way of eating.

These diets have been promoted by alternative medicine practitioners, who propose that such diets treat or prevent cancer, heart disease, low energy levels, and other illnesses. Human blood is maintained between pH 7.35 and 7.45 by acid-base homeostasis mechanisms. Levels above 7.45 are referred to as alkalosis and levels below 7.35 as acidosis. Both are potentially serious. The idea that these diets can materially affect blood pH for the purpose of treating a range of diseases is not supported by scientific research and makes incorrect assumptions about how alkaline diets function that is contrary to human physiology.

While diets avoiding meat, poultry, cheese, and grains can be used in order to make the urine more alkaline (higher pH), difficulties in effectively predicting the effects of these diets have led to medications, rather than diet modification, as the preferred method of changing urine pH. The "acid-ash" hypothesis was once considered a risk factor for osteoporosis, though the current weight of scientific evidence does not support this hypothesis.

CHAPTER:-1
ALKALINE DIET BENEFITS

There have been numerous people claiming that you can use an alkaline diet for weight loss. Is this really true? Can a person really begin to experience weight loss simply from changing their diet to consume more alkaline foods? But why is an alkaline great for weight loss? Well, a myriad of benefits has been attributed to maintaining your bodies natural pH. Reversing the effects of chronic diseases such as diabetes, heartburn, angina, migraines, and arthritis are a few of the major benefits. Freeing diabetics from their insulin crazed hunger fits has resulted in a large amount of weight loss. But, you'll see that even normal people have seen great weight loss as a result of an alkaline diet. When the body is freed of its toxic state, your metabolism is able to function more efficiently. Fat and proteins are burned and stored properly. Also, people have seen the benefits of increased energy and sex drive, allowing them to be more active and productive.

Optimizing Your Alkaline Diet for Weight Loss

If you are attempting to use an alkaline diet for weight loss, it is very important you know how to take a balanced approach. If you use alkaline water and alkaline foods in conjunction with a healthy lifestyle you will receive the "miracle" weight loss that everyone is raving about. Once you begin drinking the alkaline water on a regular basis, you can move from drinking water with pH 9.0 to pH 9.5 (for adults). Consuming a healthy amount of this high pH water is guaranteed to aid the body in returning to acid-alkaline harmony. Also, you should use the high pH water when preparing foods like soup and stews, to balance the acidifying animal proteins or other acidic aspects of the food.In the above, you have seen how you can use an alkaline diet for weight loss, but there is much more to be learned. In order to ensure that you are going to lose weight, it is important you learn about alkaline foods. Some of the most acid filled foods would be the ones you least expect. Many dairy products, for example, are very high in acid content.

Alkaline Diet for Weight Loss Tips and Benefits You Have to Know

Excessive acidic foods lead to an 'acid ash' which can be nullified through an alkaline diet. Alkaline diets are not like other diets as it concentrates on the effects food have on the acidity and alkalinity of the body.

By eating more alkaline foods, the PH of the body is not only adjusted, but it also helps with weight loss. Most diets only give short term weight loss benefits, where many people end up gaining the weight back once they are off the diet. Alkaline diets induce slow weight loss through a lifestyle change where the weight is not easily gained back.

By following an alkaline diet you have renewed energy, feel light and refreshed, get sound sleep, a slimmer body, fair skin, and an active mind. These benefits and tips should give you more reason to follow an alkaline diet for weight loss.

An alkaline diet involves the removal of acidifying foods which are high in fat and calories to induce natural and healthy weight loss. These foods include alcohol, fatty foods, red meat, high dairy products like whole milk and cheese, sugar and soda. Once you stop eating them, your body is healthier, less acidic and you start losing weight.

Most people who follow an alkaline diet for weight loss reasons also experience increased energy levels, resistance to illness and improved health and well-being. Most people take artificial sweeteners to lose weight thinking they have fewer calories than ordinary sugar.

However artificial sugars are more acidic and add toxins to your body. A better option is the moderate use of ordinary table sugar.

Many people also avoid drinking water thinking it makes them bloat. However, you need to drink lots of water as it helps wash off unwanted fats and acids from the body. It does not bloat you as it is excreted through your urine. Water is better than coffee, artificial juices with lots of water and acidic in nature and soda. Drinking alkaline water is an even better option.

Keep a big bowl of salad always ready to munch on when you come home hungry. Instead of munching on junk foods, chocolates, and instant foods in the fridge, this salad not only makes you feel full and satisfied, but its also healthy. So prepare a big serving of salad and keep it in the fridge to munch on instead of binging on unhealthy and acid rich foods.

Always keep cut vegetables and soaked nuts ready to eat in the fridge. They are a healthier option for you than an unhealthy snack and processed foods as they help increase your body alkalinity and reduces your weight.

If reading these benefits and reasons induce you to start an alkaline diet, it's better to start the diet by making small changes instead of starting it head-on. Start by reducing the amount of sugar, fat, and meat in your diet. Instead, add more fresh fruits, vegetables and healthy fats like olive oil and almonds to your diet. With time, your tastes change and adapt so that you start enjoying an alkaline diet.

Benefits of Alkaline Diet for Diabetics

Human Body Design and Alkaline Diet

The human body is, to some degree, alkaline by design. By maintaining it alkaline we allow it to run at an ideal level. Nevertheless, millions of reactions to our metabolism yield acidic wastes as end products. When we consume an excessive amount of acid-producing foods and not enough alkaline-forming foods we aggravate the body acid intoxication. If we let this acid-wastes build-up throughout the body, a disorder known as acidosis develops over time.

Acidosis will progressively debilitate our body vital functions if we do not quickly take corrective actions. Acidosis, or body over-acidity, is, in fact, one of the leading causes of human aging. It makes our body highly vulnerable to the series of deadly degenerative chronic diseases, such as diabetes, cancer, arthritis, as well as heart diseases.

For this reason, the biggest challenge we humans have to face to protect our lives is actually to find the right way to reduce the production and to maximize the elimination of the body acidic wastes. To avoid acidosis and the age-related diseases, and to continue running at its highest level possible, our body needs a healthy lifestyle. This lifestyle should include regular exercises, balanced nutrition, a clean physical environment, and a way of living that brings the lowest stress possible. A healthy lifestyle allows our body to keep its acid waste content at the lowest level possible.

The alkaline diet, also known as the pH miracle diet, seems to fit the best design of the human body.

This is mainly because it helps neutralize the acid wastes and allows flushing them out from the body. People should look at the alkaline diet as general dietary boundaries for humans' to abide by. The persons who have particular health issues and special medical diets might better accommodate those diets to alkaline diet boundaries.

CHAPTER:-2
HEALTH BENEFIT OF ALKALINE DIET

T ake Alkaline Food for Better Health

The food that we take today is totally different from our ancestors and is completely different from what we are so accustomed to these days. How aptly said, "We are what we eat." With the advancement of technology, the types of foods we consume made us dragged along. A view at the grocery store will shock you with aisles and aisles of processed food items and animal products. With the easy availability of fast foods nowadays, there is no difficulty in finding one in our neighborhood.

Fad diets are being partly to blame for introducing whole new eating habits, this includes high-protein diets. In recent years, consumption of animal products and refined food items have increased as more and more people leave out the daily supply of fruits and vegetables in their diets.

It comes as no surprise why, these days, many people are suffering from different types of ailments and allergies such as bone diseases, heart problems, and many others. Some health experts link these diseases to the type of foods we eat. There are certain types of food that disrupt the balance in our body that, during such instances, health problems arise. If only we could modify our eating habits, it's unlikely that the prevention of diseases and restoration of health can be achieved.

Why Alkaline Is Important For Our Body

For a healthy body, the alkaline and acid ration must be balanced, which is measured by the pH level in the body. pH values range from 0 to 14 and 7 is considered neutral. Any value less than 7 is considered acidic. Refined food, such as meat and meat derivatives, candies and some sweetened drinks usually generate a great amount of acid for the body.

Acidosis, a case of a high level of acidic in the bloodstream and body cells is the common index for the current different diseases inflicting many people. Some health professional's conclude that acidosis is responsible for the critical diseases suffered by many individuals nowadays.

The alkaline or alkaline diet, which normally presents in our body neutralize the high level of acidic in the body to achieve an equilibrium state. This is the main function of the alkaline in the body. However, the presence of the alkaline in the body is quickly depleted due to the high level of acidic contents it has to neutralize and there is insufficient alkaline food consumed to replenish the loss alkaline.

A Balance Alkaline-Acid Level fora Healthy Body

The good news is that while we may have subjected our bodies to years of acid abuse; abuse that is coming to light as increased infections and chronic fatigue; we can undo the damage by bringing the body's pH balance back into alignment. Optimum health is a delicate balancing act, but with practice, all of us can learn to walk the wire.

As described previously, acidosis causes many health-related problems. Critical level of acid gets into our system, breaking the cells and organs when not neutralize properly.

To prevent this, one must see to it that a balanced pH is maintained. To test whether our body contains a higher level of alkaline can be carried out with ease. This with the use of pH strips which are obtainable from any pharmacy. There are two types of strips, one for the saliva and the other for urine.

Generally, a saliva pH level strip will determine the level of acid your body is producing; the normal values should be between 6.5 and 7.5 throughout the day. A urine pH level strip will show the level of acid; a normal reading should be between 6.0 and 6.5 in the morning and between 6.5 and 7.0 at night

High Level of Acidity Is Harmful to the Body

If you consistently suffer from fatigue, headaches and having regular common cold and flu, these symptoms indicate a high level of acid in the body. The effect of acidosis in the body not only inhibits the normal diseases that we know but other diseases that you may suffer is caused by a high level of acid in the body.

Depression, high acidity, ulcer, dry skin, acne, and overweight are some of those linked with the extreme level of acidity in our body. Not limited to these, other critical and serious diseases such as joint diseases, osteoporosis, bronchitis, frequent infections, and heart diseases.

Even with medications, the symptoms may be disguised and continue to affect your health as the root of the problem has not been completely eradicated. Taking more medicine will only compound the problem as anti-inflammatory medicine will add to the acidic level in the body.

Alkaline Diet - A Sure Bet To A Healthy Body

In order to reach the root of the diseases, our systems pH value must be maintained in a healthy state. Naturally occurring alkaline foods are able to supplement the lost alkaline levels in the body during the neutralizing process. By maintaining a healthy alkaline diet, sufficient amount of alkaline is replenished in the system thereby bringing the body back to the predominant alkaline state.

So what are the ways to include an alkaline diet into our eating habits? The very basic first step is to reduce the amount of refined food intake. As we already know, these foods contain many chemicals which are the culprits in increasing the acidic level in our body. The next step is to cut down on the intake of meat and their derivatives and also the amount of liquor. The final step is to increase the number of fresh fruits and vegetables, as they are naturally high in alkalinity Oranges and lemons known for being acidic convert into alkaline after digestion and absorbed by the body is a good alkaline diet. Generally, we must consume 75% of alkaline food daily. The higher the number of alkaline foods we put into our system, the greater the neutralization of the acidic condition in our body.

What Are the Benefits of Alkaline Diets?

Wondering about the benefits of alkaline diets? Then you're not alone, because many people would love to learn more about this healthy way of eating, but they just aren't certain where to begin learning the real deal. That's why I'm giving you a guide to help you learn the truth about what alkaline diets are and the advantages that you can enjoy.

This nutrition program is called several different names, including the acid alkaline diet, the alkaline diet, and the alkaline ash diet. These names all refer to the same basic concepts, which stress fresh vegetables, fruits, whole grains, legumes, and healthy oils.

CHAPTER:-3
THE ALKALINE DIET MYTH

The alkaline dietis also known as the acid-alkaline diet or the alkaline ash diet. It is based around the idea that the foods you eat leave behind an "ash" residue after they have been metabolized. This ash can be acid or alkaline.

Proponents of this diet claim that certain foods can affect the acidity and alkalinity of bodily fluids, including urine and blood. If you eat foods with acidic ash, they make the body acidic. If you eat foods with alkaline ash, they make the body alkaline.

Acid ash is thought to make you vulnerable to diseases such as cancer, osteoporosis, and muscle wasting, whereas alkaline ash is considered to be protective. To make sure you stay alkaline, it is recommended that you keep track of your urine using handy pH test strips.

For those who do not fully understand human physiology and are not nutrition experts, diet claims like this sound rather convincing. However, is it really true? The following will debunk this myth and clear up some confusion regarding the alkaline diet.

But first, it is necessary to understand the meaning of the pH value. Put simply, the pH value is a measure of how acidic or alkaline something is. The pH value ranges from 0 to 14.

- 0-7 is acidic

- 7 is neutral

- 7-14 is alkaline

For example, the stomach is loaded with highly acidic hydrochloric acid, a pH value between 2 and 3.5. The acidity helps kill germs and break down food.

On the other hand, human blood is always slightly alkaline, with a pH of between 7.35 to 7.45. Normally, the body has several effective mechanisms (discussed later) to keep the blood pH within this range. Falling out of it is very serious and can be fatal.

Effects of Foods on Urine and Blood pH

Foods leave behind an acid or alkaline ash. Acid ash contains phosphate and sulfur. Alkaline ash contains calcium, magnesium, and potassium.

Certain food groups are considered acidic, neutral, or alkaline.

Acidic:

Meats, fish, dairy, eggs, grains, and alcohol.

Neutral:

Fats, starches, and sugars.

Alkaline:

Fruits, vegetables, nuts, and legumes.

Urine pH

Foods you eat change the pH of your urine. If you have a green smoothie for breakfast, your urine, in a few hours, will be more alkaline than if you had bacon and eggs.

For someone on an alkaline diet, urine pH can be very easily monitored and may even provide instant gratification. Unfortunately, urine pH is neither a good indicator of the overall pH of the body nor is it a good indicator of general health.

Blood pH

Foods you eat do not change your blood pH. When you eat something with acid ash like protein, the acids produced are quickly neutralized by bicarbonate ions in the blood. This reaction produces carbon dioxide, which is exhaled through the lungs, and salts, which are excreted by the kidneys in your urine.

During the process of excretion, the kidneys produce new bicarbonate ions, which are returned to the blood to replace the bicarbonate that was initially used to neutralize the acid. This creates a sustainable cycle in which the body is able to maintain the pH of the blood within a tight range.

Therefore, as long as your kidneys are functioning normally, your blood pH will not be influenced by the foods you eat, whether they are acidic or alkaline. The claim that eating alkaline foods will make your body or blood pH more alkaline is not true.

Alkaline Ionized Water Works at the Cellular Level to Promote Better Health and Healing Naturally

The Ionized water unit is projected to be the next major appliance on everyone's kitchen counter in the coming years. Why? Because what we are currently drinking is contaminated, polluted with chemicals, highly acidic and it is not conducive to promoting good health at the cellular level- and definitely not natural healing. The Japanese have been drinking a miracle liquid for 35 years that has allowed them to experience such good fortune that they rank number one in life expectancy of all nations according to the UN (United Nations) and WHO (World Health Organization). What is their secret? They drink a substance that penetrates every cell of their bodies, creating the ultimate alkaline balance, while super-hydrating and detoxifying them with every drink. It also provides them with an abundance of oxygen and more antioxidants than green tea or any supplement or food available.

Ionized water is unlike any other because it mimics the most natural and healthy water on earth found only high in the mountains - unpolluted and untainted by chemicals, preservatives or pesticides. In its natural form, it flows down the mountains and over rocks, picking up life-giving properties such as oxygen and natural alkalizing minerals from the earth. When a substance becomes alkaline it also becomes an antioxidant, which everyone knows are very good for you and help you fight illness, disease and the aging process. This process of water bouncing off of rocks and natural elements also creates a unique structure to the water molecule making the molecule clusters smaller so that it penetrates your cells and makes it easier for your body to absorb.

Smaller water molecule clusters, which also contain an abundance of stable oxygen, allows your body to experience super-hydration at the cellular level, which then allows you to flush your cells and detoxify them efficiently.

When your cells are clean, they are able to absorb nutrients and minerals which can lead to better health and a feeling of well-being. The disease cannot thrive in an environment that is alkaline and full of clean oxygen. It thrives in an acidic, dehydrated, oxygen-deprived environment.

Nature has provided you with a valuable gift, that if you take care of it properly, can provide you with a long and healthy life. Your body has the ability to naturally heal itself if given the right tools- it renews itself approximately every seven years. Depending on how healthy your cells are, depends on how well this renewal system works. If your cells are acidic, they are toxic and this will continue a cycle of mutated cells which have deformities that promote disease and premature aging.

Eating an alkaline diet can help to balance your body, by giving you extra alkaline minerals and antioxidants, but you will likely still come up short on the healing end because you still have to rid yourself of excess acids for diet alone to work effectively. Cellular health begins with proper hydration, detoxification, and oxygen that you won't get from a healthy diet alone. You are 70% water- your body's most vital substance. Without it, and unless you drink the proper amounts, you cannot hydrate properly. Water that is contaminated and polluted with chemicals only adds to more acid in your body, so you have to drink the right kind to truly battle disease and experience true health.

Why the Alkaline Diet and Cancer Is an Ideal Solution

As a result of the epidemic of cancer that has broken out in recent years, there have been great strides made in where cancer originated, how it grows in the body and how effective alkaline diet and cancer regime has become. The definition of cancer allows the patient to have some control in the prevention and battle of cancer cells.

By sticking to a primarily alkaline diet, this reduces, and actually quenches, the production of cancer and other diseases. Because of this, an alkaline diet has been found to prevent disease, while an acidic diet encourages disease and cancer to grow.

When you take the definition of cancer simply, it is 'a malformed cell.' This malformed cell can only reproduce malformed cells, and since the human body reproduces tens of thousands of cells daily, the answer is to stop that reproduction. The best defense then is a good offense, and that is

17

what an alkaline diet does as it feeds the good cells, while choking out the disease.

The foods that are taken into the body typically come from two categories - foods that produce an acidic environment and foods that produce a alkaline environment. If you are taking a large number of medicines, this might cause your system to lean more towards the acidic, but it can be counteracted by consuming more alkaline-producing foods.

A alkaline diet is generally made up of alkaline-producing foods so that the pH level is brought to an level of around 7.4. If you search online there are alkaline/acidic charts of all the foods. If you are just beginning this diet, make a copy of the chart and carry it with you when you shop or go out to eat. In general, stay away from processed foods, fast foods fried in trans fat, any food made with white sugar or white flour, and all foods with chemicals and steroids. These foods all feed cancer cells. If this is what your diet is made up of, check the alkaline food list and see what to be eating now.

Foods on that are alkaline-producing are vegetables, seeds, most fruits, brown rice, and other grains, and fish.

These foods can be mixed and matched to your own preference for at least 80% of your total diet, and then you add 20% of the acidic-producing foods, and the acidic foods are not all "bad". Foods on the acidic side are whole grain bread, lean meats, milk, and milk products, butter and eggs, and this adds up to make a 100% alkaline diet.

To monitor your pH level once you have gotten started on an alkaline diet and cancer-fighting way of eating, check any health food store for pH strips or litmus paper. There will be a color chart included to use and determine what your pH blood level is. For an alkaline system, it should register between 7.2 - 7.8. No two people are alike, so test your pH level about once a day as you get started. Then continue to check once a week. If you need to raise your pH level, eat more alkaline foods and use green supplements. An alkaline diet will prevent disease naturally.

Acidic Diet and Cancer

Those who advocate an alkaline diet claim that it can cure cancer because cancer can only grow in an acidic environment. By eating an alkaline diet, cancer cells cannot grow but die.

This hypothesis is very flawed. Cancer is perfectly capable of growing in an alkaline environment. In fact, cancer grows in normal body tissue which has a slightly alkaline pH of 7.4. Many experiments have confirmed this by successfully growing cancer cells in a alkaline environment.

However, cancer cells to grow faster with acidity. Once a tumor starts to develop, it creates its own acidic environment by breaking down glucose and reducing circulation. Therefore, it is not the acidic environment that causes cancer but cancer that causes the acidic environment.

Even more interesting is a 2005 study by the National Cancer Institute which uses vitamin C (ascorbic acid) to treat cancer. They found that by administering pharmacologic doses intravenously, ascorbic acid successfully killed cancer cells without harming normal cells. This is another example of cancer cells being vulnerable to acidity, as opposed to alkalinity.

In short, there is no scientific link between eating an acidic diet and cancer. Cancer cells can grow in both acidic and alkaline environments.

Acidic Diet and Osteoporosis

Osteoporosis is a progressive bone disease characterized by a decrease in bone mineral content, leading to lowered bone density and strength and a higher risk of a broken bone.

Proponents' of the alkaline diet believe that in order to maintain a constant blood pH, the body takes alkaline minerals like calcium from the bones to neutralize the acids from an acidic diet. As discussed above, this is absolutely not true. The kidneys and the respiratory system are responsible for regulating blood pH, not the bones.

In fact, many studies have shown that increasing animal protein intake is positive for bone metabolism as it increases calcium retention and activates IGF-1 (insulin-like growth factor-1) that stimulates bone regeneration. Thus, the hypothesis that an acidic diet causes bone loss is not supported by science.

Acidic Diet and Muscle Wasting

Advocates of the alkaline diet believe that in order to eliminate excess acid caused by an acidic diet, the kidneys will steal amino acids (building blocks of protein) from muscle tissues, leading to muscle loss. The proposed mechanism is similar to the one causing osteoporosis.

As discussed, blood pH is regulated by the kidneys and the lungs, not the muscles. Hence, acidic foods like meats, dairy, and eggs do not cause muscle loss. As a matter of fact, they are complete dietary proteins that will support muscle repair and help prevent muscle wasting.

What Did Our Ancestors Eat?

A number of studies have examined whether our pre-agricultural ancestors ate net acidic or net alkaline diets. Very interestingly, they found that about half of the hunter-gatherers ate net acid-forming diets, while the other half ate net alkaline-forming diets.

Acid-forming diets were more common as people moved further north of the equator. The less hospitable the environment, the more animal proteins they ate. In more tropical environments where fruits and vegetables were abundant, their diet became more alkaline.

From an evolutionary perspective, the theory that acidic or protein-rich diets cause diseases like cancer, osteoporosis, and muscle loss is not valid. Half of the hunter-gatherers were eating net acid-forming diets, yet, they had no evidence of such degenerative diseases.

It is worth noting that there is no one-size-fits-all diet that works for everyone, which is why Metabolic Typing is so helpful in determining your optimal diet. Due to our genetic variances, some people will benefit from an acidic diet, some an alkaline diet, and some in between. Thus the saying: one man's food can be another man's poison.

. Eating fewer grains will benefit those who are gluten-sensitive or have leaky gut or an autoimmune disease.

CHAPTER:-4
ALKALINE WATER

O ne last point worth mentioning is that many people believe that drinking alkaline water (pH of 9.5 vs. pure water's pH of 7.0.) is healthier based on similar reasoning as the alkaline diet. Anyhow, it is not true. Water that is too alkaline can be detrimental to your health and lead to nutritional disequilibrium.

If you drink alkaline water all the time, it will neutralize your stomach acid and raise the alkalinity of your stomach. Over time, it will impair your ability to digest food and absorb nutrients and minerals. With less acidity in the stomach, it will also open the door for bacteria and parasites to get into your small intestine.

The bottom line is that alkaline water is not the answer to good health. Do not be fooled by marketing gimmicks. Instead, invest in a good water filtration system for your home. Clean, filtered water is still the best water for your body.

Carol Chuang is a Certified Nutrition Specialist and a Metabolic Typing Advisor. She has a Masters degree in Nutrition and is the founder of CC Health Counseling, LLC. Her passion in life is to stay healthy and to help others become healthy. She believes that a key ingredient to optimal health is to eat a diet that is right for one's specific body type. Eating organic or eating healthy is not enough to guarantee good health. The truth is that there is no one diet that is right for everyone. Our metabolisms are different, so should our diets.

Can an Alkaline Diet Help Prevent Osteoporosis?

It can be quite scary to get the news. "I am sorry to tell you, ma'am. You have osteoporosis". No one wants to be sitting in that chair hearing that news. All over North American, thousands of women and even men are hearing it though. The thought of not being able to enjoy life anymore because of the risk of having a un-healable bone break is scary, to say the least.

First of all, this condition seems to affect the women and men of North America more than other countries. In fact, in Asia, it is quite rare for women to get osteoporosis. Some other startling facts include:

1. It is NOT normal for one's bones to get more brittle as we age. Bone metabolism is set up to keep our bones strong for our entire lives.

2. It is NOT just a female condition. Men also are showing signs of this condition

3. It is NOT just a condition of the elderly. More and more, younger patients are being diagnosed with this condition

4. It is NOT caused by low calcium intake

5. It is NOT only caused by the effect of lowered estrogen production

What Dr. Brown goes on to show in her book is the total effect of one's lifestyle on your bone strength.

Your diet, your stress levels, and your physical activity all go hand in hand to determine your bone strength. The typical SAD diet (Standard American Diet) is partly to blame for this condition. In addition, a lack of physical activity as we older only makes things worse.

So, want are people to do to avoid becoming another osteoporosis statistic? First, learn about the acid-alkaline balance in your body. The foods we eat, external stress in our lives, physical stress, all add to the acidity of our body. Most importantly, the acidic level of our blood is of primary concern. If the blood becomes too acidic, the chemical processes that occur inside our cells stop. Taking this to the extreme, the body will die. So, to prevent this, the body has a mechanism of controlling the acid level. It does this with acid-buffering minerals such as calcium, magnesium, potassium, sodium, chromium, Selenium, and iron.

These best source of these minerals in our body is our bones. As the body works to overcome an over-acidic condition, it will do so at the sake of our bones, leading to poor bone density. To prevent this from happening, and to even reverse it, you should consider adopting an alkaline diet. Most green plants and sprouts are very alkaline. Foods that are high in sugars, proteins, refined foods, alcohols, and starches are acid forming. Dr. Brown calls these antinutrients. In the book, we are told to avoid excessive protein, reduce our caffeine consumption, eliminate sugars and excessive fats, reduce our salt intake and avoid alcohol and tobacco products. Next, replace all of these antinutrients with alkaline foods. This may be challenging for some people and the promise is that once your body is in balance, you could never consider going back to your old eating habits. The pleasure of being in acid-alkaline balance will overcome any cravings you may 'think' you will have.

We have long known the benefits of regular exercise.

When combined with an alkaline diet, however, a daily physical fitness program, including strength training can go a long way to helping prevent

Osteoporosis.

This treatise has been an introduction to the things you can do to stop this condition before it starts. It is not a replacement for sound medical advice. To obtain recommendations appropriate for your current situation, always seek the counsel of a qualified health care provider.

Alkaline Diet Guidelines For Osteoporosis Treatment

An alkaline diet that emphasizes lots of fruits and vegetables is generally considered the best diet for the prevention and treatment of osteoporosis. Unfortunately, this is not the diet that is familiar to most North Americans.

The North American Diet

There is a growing consensus that a good diet for osteoporosis will avoid excessive acid-forming foods and beverages such as meat, soft drinks, and coffee. In "Strategies for Osteoporosis", the National Osteoporosis Foundation warns that excessive protein consumption can be damaging to bone health. "Excessive protein and sodium intake can increase calcium loss through the kidneys. In fact, an individual's daily calcium requirement increases in direct proportion to the amount of protein and sodium in his/her diet."

The Institute of Arthritis and Musculoskeletal and Skin Diseases (NIAMS) repeats this warning: "Although a balanced diet aids calcium absorption, high levels of protein and sodium (salt) in the diet are thought to increase calcium excretion through the kidneys. Excessive amounts of these substances should be avoided, especially in those with low calcium intake." North American consumption of meat and soda beverages may be a partial cause of the high incidence of osteoporosis relative to other countries.

Meat the Recommended Dietary Allowance (RDA) of protein for men is 56 grams/day and for women 46 grams/day from all food sources including meat, tofu, eggs, grains, legumes, and dairy products.

Statistics Canada reports that Canadian consumption of red meat (including beef, pork, mutton, and veal) and chicken has been slowly declining since 1999 to approximately 77 pounds (35 kg) per person in 2007 or 25 grams of protein a day. (This calculation is for meat only and does not include other protein-rich foods such as dairy products.) Meat consumption may be declining in Canada but it is steadily increasing in the U.S. to an extraordinary 101 kg (223 pounds) per capita in 2007-or 72 grams of protein a day from meat alone...not including eggs, dairy, grain or legumes. As this includes every man, woman, and child, adults are clearly consuming far more than the recommended level of animal protein.

Soft Drinks & Coffee

Medical research has also identified a clear link between cola and osteoporosis -but again in the United States, soft drink consumption continues to increase along with the demand for more meat

A study conducted at the University of North Carolina at Chapel Hill showed that energy intake from soft drinks in the United States increased 135 percent between about 1977 and 2001. Young adult's ages 19 to 39 drank the softest drinks, increasing their intake from 4.1 percent to 9.8 percent of total daily calorie consumption during that period. Among coffee drinkers (i.e. not per capita) the average coffee consumption in the United States is 3.1 cups of coffee per day (National Coffee Association) and consumption is also increasing.

According to Agriculture and Agri-Food Canada, per capita consumption of soft drinks in Canada has declined during the past decade but was still almost 110 liters per capita in 2006. Soft drinks still hold the largest market share of all beverages that are sold (15%) although coffee consumption is increasing and was over 14% of the beverage market in 2006. Together these two acid producing drinks comprise almost 30% of beverages consumed by Canadians. Research now suggests that people who are trying to follow alkaline diet guidelines for osteoporosis prevention or treatment should avoid cola drinks and drink decaffeinated coffee if they can't live without their java. An even healthier choice would be to reduce meat consumption in favor of fruits and vegetables and drink non-caffeinated drinks such as green tea.

We do not have to become vegetarians to comply with alkaline diet guidelines for osteoporosis treatment. But reducing our soda and meat consumption and increasing vegetables and fruit in our diet is definitely indicated. A general rule-of-thumb is to have a diet consisting of 20% acid-forming foods (grains and protein) and 80% alkaline-forming foods (fruits and vegetables). An healthy goal would be to include at least two vegetable or fruit servings at every meal and to eat no more than two daily servings of carbs such as bread, cereal, and pasta.

Choosing Alkaline Diets Is The Only Way To Live A Healthy Lifestyle

The low carbohydrate and high protein diets doing the rounds these days are an invitation to bad health. All athletes know that if a fit body is to be maintained one should steer completely clear of such diets. Not only do they result in extreme fatigue but also are a disaster where weight management is concerned. Choosing alkaline diets is the only way to live a healthy life as well as shed those extra pounds.

Alkaline diets require one to follow a lifestyle completely opposite of the high protein low carb diets. The high protein diets leave the person following it fatigued and tired. It is for those who lead a stagnant life and want to shed some weight. But the weight that is lost comes back on as soon as one stops the diet. With alkaline diets, this is not the case. The diets can be incorporated into one's way of life and within days the results start to show. They require one to eat about 80 % alkalizing foods so as to maintain the alkaline ph of the body to 7.4. High protein diets tend to make the ph of the body acidic as opposed to its natural alkaline tilt. When the body ph becomes acidic it attracts all illnesses and depletes one of energy. An acidic ph also results in rapid degeneration of the human body cells. That leads to a shortened life. One should stay away from these crash diets and look at achieving health and vigor by following alkaline diets instead.

Alkaline diets lead to the body ph maintaining its alkaline nature. The various body functions are carried out smoothly and the immune system of the body stays strong. Under these circumstances, one feels energetic as opposed to feeling fatigued. Also, the weight shed like this stays off and most importantly the body does not fall sick. In other words, they help repel diseases as opposed to high protein diets which seem to attract them.

These plans are also very good for those suffering from chronic diseases like arthritis, cancer, migraines, sinusitis and also osteoporosis. Following such a regime while taking medication helps fight these diseases off from the root.

Alkaline diets constitute mostly of fruits and vegetables. One should try and consume green vegetables and sweet fruits so that they make up about 70 to 80 percent of their total food intake. Lemons and melons should also be eaten. Almonds, honey, and olive oil are also high on the list of foods to be consumed for following alkaline diets. Meats and fats should be avoided. All foods that are acidifying like coffee, alcohol, meats and even certain vegetables like cooked spinach should not form more than 20% of one's diet. Alkaline water is also a must for everyone wanting to improve their diet. At least 6 to 8 glasses of alkaline water can do wonders for your body cleansing. Processed food is all acidic and also high on weight gaining substances and so should be avoided. Beverages like sodas are highly acidic and should not be consumed at all. It takes 32 glasses of water to balance out one glass of soda.

Alkaline diets are for everyone. Each one of us should stop abusing our bodies and look at a healthy and long life by making alkaline diets a part of our lifestyle.

CHAPTER:-5
ACID TO ALKALINE DIET

What Is an Acid Alkaline Diet?

A lot of people have been struggling to find the best diet program fit for them. One of the most common misrepresentation that these people have is their desire to lose weight. They fail to put vital emphasis on how to be healthy. If you want to know the best diet that is perfect for you, then you better make sure its healthy and is not destroying your body.

The acid to alkaline diet is becoming more talked about subject nowadays but still, the majority of the population are unaware of what it is. People who die young, have health problems, suffer from obesity, etc., generally, have a very acidic internal environment whereas people who live to very old age and don't suffer from serious health problems have an internal environment that is more alkaline in nature.

In the modern Western world, the vast majority of people live a very unhealthy lifestyle, predominantly eating junk and unhealthy food and being constantly exposed to other factors that drastically impact our health in a negative way, in drastic contrast to the acid to the alkaline diet. According to the World Health Organization (WHO), there are more that one billion obese adults worldwide, with around 300 million of them clinically obese. This statistic is scary and is dramatically increasing every day!

As a health care practitioner myself, people often ask me what are the best ways to stay healthy. I often tell my patients that in order for us to live a healthy life, not be overweight, avoid serious disease and illnesses and generally live to a good old age with vitality and vigor, it is essential that we pay attention to the acid to the alkaline diet.

By observing your bodies pH levels and eating accordingly to ensure your body is more alkaline than acidic, people experience things like rapid weight loss (by an accelerated fat disposal process), they will live longer, feel less stressed, have an improved immune system, get better and more restful sleep, have more energy and can also experience an increase in libido.

These benefits alone are of course of tremendous importance to health, longevity and happy life. By allowing the body to detox in this way through the acid to alkaline diet people also have an increased ability to absorb vitamins and minerals and help avoid many nasty diseases including cancer and arthritis. With a more alkaline body, stress and pressure on the internal organs are eased, skin, bones, and cells regenerate and help keep you youthful.

Conversely, if a person's body is too acidic they can easily experience obesity by gaining and holding onto fat, they will age quicker, a lack of energy will be common, they will easily and consistently attract disease and virus' and create an internal environment where yeast and bacteria can easily thrive.

The majority of people living in the Western world don't follow an acid to an alkaline diet and are generally more on the acidic scale.

This is due largely to our diet. Eating things like junk food, burgers, fizzy drinks, having a high sugar intake, fried foods, unnatural fruit juices, imitation foods, energy drinks, and processed foods, for example, all push our bodies internal environment down on the acidic scale.

There are even some otherwise healthy foods to be aware of, strawberries, mangos, and peaches, for example, are very high in sugar, therefore create an acidic environment in the body. Some other surprises that also cause the acidic build up to include rice, tuna, oats, and cheese, so these foods are to be limited when following an acid to the alkaline diet.

This is one reason why it is very important to know exactly what foods will cause an acid reaction and which will make you more alkaline. Other considerations that also cause our bodies to be more acidic include various chemicals, tobacco, radiation, pesticides, artificial sweeteners, air pollution, alcohol, drugs, and stress.

Optimal pH to get all the benefits from alkalinity is 7.4pH. If your body goes 3-4 points either way you will die! The pH scale is as follows:

0 = total acid/battery acid, hydrochloric acid

1 = gastric juices

2 = vinegar

3 = beer

4 = wine, tomato juice

5 = rain

6 = milk

7 = pure water

8 = sea water

9 = baking soda

10 = detergent, milk of magnesia

11 = ammonia, lime water

12 = bleach

13 = lye

14 = Total Alkaline/Sodium Hydroxide

The acid to the alkaline diet will help your body stay at the optimal range, around 7.4pH. The bodies reaction to trying to keep this acid, alkaline balance is both incredible and fascinating. When your body is too acidic it tries everything to get to a more alkaline state.

When this happens the body stores some acid in your fat to keep it from doing harm to our body which is a good thing, but your body then holds on to the fat for protection, causing the person to put on weight.

When there is excess acid internally, the body finds alkaline elsewhere from your bones and teeth but your bones and teeth get so drained that they become frail and start to decay. This can lead to many diseases of the bones and teeth including arthritis and tooth decay. This would not happen if a person were following an acid to an alkaline diet.

The build-up of an acid generally will settle away from your healthier organs but instead, it gravitates towards your weakest organs that are already prone to disease. It's like a pack of wolves looking for the weakest amongst the herd, picking off the easy prey.

As your weaker organs are targeted it makes it much easier for serious diseases to set in, including cancer. It is important to realize that cancer cells become dormant if you are at 7.4pH (which is the bodies optimum pH levels), thus further underlining the importance of maintaining a healthy pH level in our bodies by following the acid to the alkaline diet.

When there is acid in the system it also contaminates your bloodstream. This, in turn, prevents the type's of blood ability to deliver oxygen to the tissues. RBC's are surrounded by a negative charge so they can bounce off each other and move around in the blood very quickly and deliver their best. But when you are too acidic they lose their negative charge and they stick together, causing them to move very slowly.

CHAPTER:-6
REAL DEAL WITH ALKALINE DIET

T his causes them to struggle to deliver nutrients and oxygen in our system. One of the first symptoms of this poisoning is you start to feel a loss of energy even though you are getting enough sleep. Starting an acid to an alkaline diet can correct this very quickly. Your blood also has this reaction after drinking alcohol.

Let's put all this into perspective; it takes about 33 glasses of water to neutralize one glass of coke! I'm not even going to mention here what it takes to neutralize some of the other things that we are putting into our bodies, I think you get the picture!

One great way to consistently make your body more alkaline is by having green drinks every day. They are very easy to make, taste great and are packed with vitamins, minerals, and chlorophyll which fuel our body. Chlorophyll is a big part of the acid to an alkaline diet and is the green blood of plants.

It is a very powerful detoxify-er, blood builder, cleaner and oxygen booster. In fact, the benefits of chlorophyll on our bodies are far too numerous to include in this article. There are many recipes for making tasty green drinks. The one I am currently having every day is as follows; 2 apples, 4 sticks celery, 1/3 cucumber, a big handful of baby spinach leaves and one avocado. I have been doing this every day (more or less) for about the last six months and not once have I been sick. I have also noticed an increase in energy and I am also benefiting from more restful sleep.

Alkaline Diet: Acidic and Alkaline Foods

Gastric hyperacidity is one of the most common medical conditions.

Furthermore, metabolic acidosis is said to be the basis of all disease, since it is directly related to various kidney problems, to diabetes, ulcer and many other internal diseases.

Therefore, the purpose of the alkaline diet is to bring the pH to normal and also to help people lose weight, not through caloric deficit, but by replacing some other acidic foods with alkaline foods.

The alkaline diet is a modern one which was born from the desire/need for people to treat gastric hyperacidity and prevent or postpone as many problems caused by acidosis.

Alkaline Diet plan involves creating a compound food as follows:

a.75% alkaline foods, which have a pH greater than 7.4, as close to 8;

b. 25% acidic foods;

What is the difference between acidic foods and those for the alkaline diet?

In terms of chemical, acidic foods are saturated with hydrogen ions, while the alkaline has a chemical structure that allows the absorption of hydrogen ions.

Normally, the internal pH (of blood) is 7.38 to 7, 52. It is vital that the pH does not drop below 7, as this may induce grade IV coma and even death of the patient. Also, the blood does not have to have a very basic character, but only slightly alkaline, otherwise there is the risk of involuntary muscle contractions, extremely powerful and painful.

Foods Are Alkaline And Which Are Acidic?

In the acidic food category, there are all traditional foods, sodas, pastries and of course, alcoholic beverages. Chicken, beef, turkey, pasta, refined oil, pickles (very acidic!), all cookies and all derivatives of the above products have a relatively high acidity, whose value may rise or fall in depending on the mode of preparation.

In the alkaline diet foods category we have:

a. Cottage cheese, cucumbers and lettuce, avocado and all the vegetables and edible plants rich in chlorophyll;

b. Soya milk, soya chunks, coconut, lemon, millet, beans, and buckwheat;

c.Seabuckthorn;

d.Cold pressed oil of any kind;

Alkaline water is vital for alkaline diet!

For those who can not maintain the recommended percentage in the diet (75% alkaline foods and 25% acidic foods), it is recommended to replace drinks with alkaline water. Any water that has a pH greater than 7.7 is considered alkaline water and can be consumed in large quantities. The risk of blood pH to increase to critical values is very low, 2.5-3 liters of alkaline water a day should help anyone to maintain its optimum health and always help detoxify the body and cleaning of free radicals.

Smoking is prohibited!

Smoking is a habit that grows very much acidity in the body, which happens when we drink alcohol too.

Acid Alkaline Diet Benefits & Why It Is Recommended

If you have heard of the Atkins diet, then the Acid Alkaline Diet is the complete opposite of that. The Atkins diet is a high protein, high fat but low carbohydrates diet. But such diets have a tendency to leave one low on energy and also they seem to be improper gastronomically speaking.

An acid alkaline diet, on the other hand, is not only useful for weight loss but over an above, that is extremely beneficial to the body functioning. An Acid-alkaline, also known as an alkaline ash diet, alkaline acid diet, and the alkaline diet, keeps the ph level of the body balanced and so safeguards against various illnesses. Even chronic diseases like arthritis can be not only prevented but also cured if such a diet is followed.

The basis of a diet that is acid-alkaline lies in the fact that our body ph ideally should be a 7.3. This slightly alkaline level of the body ph keeps all the vital organs functioning well, as well as the absorption of various minerals is optimized. When this ph tilts to the acidic side trouble starts brewing. An acidic ph level leads to almost all body parts suffering in one way or the other. Now since our body needs to be alkaline in nature it should reflect in our food intake too. Foods that are alkalizing should be consumed much more as opposed to acidifying foods. Translated in a simpler language this would mean more of vegetable and fruit consumption and very low meats and oil intake.

If the body's alkaline minerals such as calcium, magnesium and potassium levels drop so will its health causing it to degenerate and its defenses to drop guard? An alkaline diet protects that from happening. An acid alkaline or an alkaline ash diet comprises of 80% alkalizing foods and 20 % acidic foods. Since the acid-alkaline ratio in the body should be one is to four our food intake should be of similar nature.

An alkaline diet is not only recommended to shed those extra pounds but is also and more importantly a great means of regaining lost health and leading longer and more diseases free life. This diet is especially recommended to those who feel tired most of the time. Stress and a low energy level can both be done away with a diet that is acid-alkaline.

Those who suffer from frequent viral fevers or those who have nasal congestion most of the time can lead healthier lives if they have a diet that is acid-alkaline. Weak nails, dryness, headaches, muscle pain, hives, joint pains, and many more such diseases find their answer in an alkaline ash diet.

An higher level of vegetable intake is recommended in an alkaline ash diet. Lemons should be squeezed into water drinks. Millet or quinoa is preferred over wheat, olive oil over vegetable oil and soups like miso are very useful for following an alkaline ash diet.

Lost health and vigor can be regained and many chronic illnesses prevented as well as cured if an acid alkaline diet is followed. It is a fairly easy diet plan, which should adopt for a longer and healthier life span.

Where Can I Find Alkaline Diet Recipes?

When you first discover the alkaline diet and its many benefits - from great levels of energy and vitality to its anti-aging properties, great digestion, disease prevention and a general uplift in health - the natural question is "Where can I find alkaline diet recipes?"

The refreshing answer is that many recipes and meals that you already know and enjoy can be made more alkaline by making some simple substitutions of foods that are alkaline.

Following the alkaline diet means swapping acidic foods like meat, dairy, refined sugars and fats, and other processed foods for alkaline foods such as vegetables, leafy greens, some fruits and nuts, and seeds.

So for example, you can make an alkaline version of spaghetti Bolognese by swapping the minced beef for brown lentils, swapping the jar of processed Bolognese tomato sauce for a home-made version containing tomatoes, herbs and spices, some flax oil, onions and a few other unprocessed, natural ingredients blended together and swapping the durum wheat spaghetti for raw courgette noodles made with a vegetable specialize.

Another fantastic alkaline diet recipe that is so good it's hard to believe it's healthy for you is alkaline banana ice cream: You simply take a bunch of over-ripe bananas, peel them, cut them up into chunks and freeze them. Then when you want to eat the ice cream, take 10 or so of the frozen chunks, blend them in your high-speed blender with a little coconut or almond milk and a teaspoon of mica (a calciferous root vegetable super-food that tastes a little malt-like) if you wish.

You could also add some vanilla extract or lucuma powder (custard-tasting super food) to make it more 'creamy'. Simple, healthy, delicious! It's truly hard to believe that this ice cream recipe has no dairy in it and the consistency is just like proper ice cream.

A question that is asked a lot is whether or not fruits are alkaline. The simple answer is that it depends: As long as fruits are eaten alone, before any other slower-digesting foods and in the context of an overall vegetable-based diet, then they complement this and help to alkalize your body. If they are not combined properly then they can ferment and cause acidification. So it's good to inform yourself about optimum food combining protocols.

A good rule of thumb for making recipes alkaline is to keep them as unprocessed as possible - raw, natural ingredients are best - and by substituting meat and dairy products for vegetables and beans, pulses and nuts and seeds.

Some simple swaps you can easily make alkalize your diet and body: Coconut milk for dairy milk; steamed vegetables for rice, pasta, and bread; pulses for meat; fruits for refined sugar products; water and herbal teas for coffee, soda, and alcohol.

Back to Basics With an Alkaline Diet

When you choose to eat an alkaline diet, you are actually eating foods that are very similar to what man was designed to eat. If you look at what our ancestors ate, you will find a diet rich in fresh fruits, vegetables, legumes, nuts, and fish. Unfortunately, man's diet today is frequently full of foods that are high in unhealthy fats, salt, cholesterol, and acidifying foods.

How Our Diet Changed

Although some people think that man's diet changed only recently, the shift from a largely alkaline diet to an acid diet actually began thousands of years ago. Our original diet consisted of foraged fruits, nuts, and vegetables, and along with whatever meat could be caught. As soon as the man started to grow his own food, things started to change. Grains became a popular diet choice, especially after the development of stone tools. Once animal's were domesticated, there were dairy products added to the diet, along with an additional amount of meat. Salt began to be added, along with sugar. The end result was a diet that was still much healthier than what many people eat today, but the shift from alkaline to acid had begun.

Recent Dietary Changes

It's no secret that our modern diet consists of many foods which are not healthy for us. Too much junk food and "fast food" has decreased the quality of our diet. Obesity has become the norm, and along with with it a higher incidence of diseases such as diabetes, coronary disease, and cancer. If you want to improve your health and reduce the risk of many diseases, an alkaline diet can help get your body back to basics.

The Alkaline Diet

Surely, you have encountered an alkaline meal program somewhere online or in some reading materials. What is an alkaline diet and is this diet healthy for you? This diet all started when experts tried considering the pH level of the body. In a person's body, the environment can be acidic or alkaline.

Once the pH level is high then the environment is alkaline. In contrary, low pH means

The environment is acidic. The body does not have one single pH level rather it can differ depending on the location. The pH level in the stomach is different from the urinary bladder.

This diet is basically all about eating foods which can promote an alkaline environment in the body while not eating foods that promote acidity to the body. What could be the reason behind this program? To start off, foods that can promote an alkaline environment in the body, are considered healthy. Examples of these foods include vegetables, fruits, soy products, nuts, legumes, and cereals. If you have noticed, these foods are rich in protein, vitamins, and minerals.

The other principle of an alkaline diet is to avoid acid foods because these are foods that can make your body at risk for weight gain, heart problems, kidney and liver diseases. Few of the many acid foods include caffeine, foods with high preservatives like canned goods, sodas, fish, meat, alcohol, and foods with high sugar content. When you come to think of it, an alkaline diet is not unusual for everyone especially when talking about a healthy diet.

According to experts, acidic foods can decrease the pH of a person's urine. When the pH is abnormally low kidney stones tend to form. To counteract this situation a person needs to increase the pH through eating alkaline rich foods, that simple.

Since an alkaline diet means avoiding alcohol and any other foods with high acidity, it also means that you will decrease the risk of developing diseases associated with an unhealthy diet like diabetes, hypertension, and obesity. Although no exact pieces of evidence can prove, some researchers have stated that the alkaline diet can reduce the risk of cancer.

Things to Remember

In order for the alkaline diet to work, you must condition yourself to adhere to the diet program. When it requires you to avoid unhealthy foods and drinks, then you better do it. Water therapy is an excellent alternative drink for soda and alcohol. In addition, so that you will not have a difficult time figuring out which are alkaline and which are acid foods, it is best that you make a list of each category. Perhaps you can research online on what foods are rich in alkaline and those having high acid content. Alkaline foods are not that hard to point because the majority of foods belong to vegetables and fruits classification.

The Alkaline Diet - What Can I Eat on It?

The Alkaline Diet is also known as the Alkaline Ash Diet, Alkaline Acid Diet, or the Acid Alkaline Diet.

Generally, the diet consists of eating certain citrus, other low sugar fruits, vegetables, tubers, nuts, and legumes.

Grains, dairy products, meat, sugar, alcohol, caffeine, and fungi like mushrooms are to be avoided. By consuming such a diet, it is said that the body maintains a pH of between 7.35 and 7.45 (7.00 is neutral on the pH scale while below 7.00 is acidic).

Diet and Disease

There is some evidence that such a diet is beneficial in preventing osteoporosis and other bone health issues. However, the evidence is not strong in supporting the claims that an alkaline diet may prevent or help alleviate conditions such as cancer, fatigue, obesity, or allergies.

There is, however, some evidence that cancer cells grow more quickly in an acidic environment in a laboratory setting. Therefore, a person with a predisposition to or who actually suffers from this disease may want to investigate the effects an alkaline diet have on the body.

Considering the overwhelming rise in many of these types of diseases it is easy to wonder if they are caused by the general condition of a person's internal body environment.

A wider and more scientifically rigorous examination of the Alkaline Diet is in order. However, such scientific scrutiny may be tainted from the beginning by prejudice fomented in a pharmaceutical-based health care delivery system.

The theory behind the Alkaline Diet is not widely accepted by the medical community which may be one of the reasons cancer, diabetes, and any number of other terrible diseases are at epidemic levels. The Alkaline Diet, when combined with a physically active, low-stress lifestyle certainly deserves more attention from the scientific community if they can keep their bias at bay.

Good Healthy Food

So, what are you supposed to eat?

It is recommended that you avoid "acidic" foods such as sugar, red meat, shellfish, eggs, dairy, processed and other refined foods, most grains including refined grains, artificial sweeteners, alcohol, caffeine, chocolate, and soda pop.

You should consume raw fruits and vegetables that have a high chlorophyll content such as green leafy vegetables. The brassica family of vegetables (also known as crucifers) are well represented on the Alkaline Diet and include:

- Broccoli

- Brussels sprouts

- Cabbage

- Cauliflower

- Turnips

- Collard greens

- Kale

- Kohlrabi

- Bok Choi

- Mustard Greens

Other raw vegetables to try on your alkaline diet are:

- Avocado

- Tomato

- Red Beets

- Carrots

- Lima Beans

- Red and black radishes

- Rutabaga

- Eggplant

- Asparagus

- Artichoke

- Lettuce

- Cucumber

- Celery

- Peppers

- Zucchini

- Squash

- Spinach

- Peas

- Parsnips

- Onions

Healthy Fruit

The best fruit to consume on the alkaline diet includes:

- Unripe bananas

- Sour cherries

- Fresh coconut

- Figs (either raw or dried)

- Fresh lemon

- Lime

Whether the Alkaline Diet is as good for preventing disease as its proponents claim will have to wait to be seen.

However, following the alkaline diet certainly will keep you within the parameters of what most other medical practitioners and organizations have been claiming to be a healthy diet for many, many years.

How to Lose Weight With an Alkaline Diet and Alkaline Foods

Those struggling with excess weight see countless advertisements of thousands of weight loss products. Yet most of these people don't even know WHY they are overweight in the first place. Many people like to have more energy throughout the day, but the snacks and caffeinated drinks that many consumers are highly acid-forming.

What Excess Acidity Does Inside The Body

By creating acidity in blood, tissue and body cells, these typical snacks (as well as fast food, processed food, sweets, all yeast containing products, etc!) may interfere with healthy energy production and often result in subsequent weight gain. The reason for that is the body's response to excess acidity: it stores acid wastes in fat cells to prevent them from vital organs.

The over-acidification / acidosis of our body cells is the reason for many diseases, will interrupt cellular activities and functions, and is what causes overweight: to protect itself from potentially serious damage, the body creates new fat cells to store the extra acid. However, as soon as the acidic environment is eliminated, the fat inside the body is no longer needed and literally melts away.

The body's internal environment is slightly alkaline, which is why it demands a diet that is also slightly alkaline. The body's entire metabolic process depends on an alkaline environment. Our internal system lives and dies at the cellular level, all the billions of cells that make up the human body are slightly alkaline, and must maintain alkalinity in order to function and remain healthy and alive.

Alkaline Food will make food cravings subside naturally because the acidity inside the internal environment is neutralized through the alkaline-forming elements. Once the inner terrain is alkalized with alkaline water and alkaline food according to an alkaline diet (=weight loss diet), the body is free to release the acid waste and burns off fat. In this way, your pH level will also be balanced, and every organ functions better, supporting healthy metabolism and making weight control much easier.

Some Good Alkaline Foods

Fresh vegetables, greens, and grasses are excellent anti-yeast and anti-fungal foods, and green grasses such as barley or wheat grass are some of the lowest-calorie, lowest-sugar and most nutrient-rich foods on earth (and contain high amounts of fiber).

Alkaline foods are mostly vegetables, especially raw ones. Most alkalizing are wheat and alfalfa grasses, fresh cucumber and some kind of sprouts. Furthermore, limes, tomatoes, and avocado also have an alkalizing effect on our body, same as most kind of seeds, tofu, fresh soybeans, almonds, or olive oil.

Discover How Alkaline Diet Recipes Whip up Better Health

In general, this diet involves ingesting certain fresh citrus fruits and food that is low in sugar it promotes to avoid food which is high in acids such as grains, dairy, meat, sugar, alcohol, caffeine, and fungi. It actually cut off the daily intake of acidic foods to a limit of 30% and boosts your alkaline intake to 70%. The goal is to limit or even eliminate the ingestion of foods which are detrimental to health and replace it with savory healthy alkaline diet recipes.

CHAPTER:-7
RESULT OF ALKALINE DIET?

O nce an alkaline diet is started, most people discover that their pH naturally becomes more alkaline. One gets to see how certain type's of meals create a very acidic environment and learn to adjust their eating habits to better support weight control. When pH balance is achieved through alkaline food and alkaline eating habits, the body naturally drops to its healthy weight, food cravings will diminish, and blood-sugar levels are balanced and energy levels will increase immensely.

So anybody who is ready to pursue the path of better health, weight loss, and more energy should consider the advantages of the alkaline diet for achieving an optimal pH balance in the body. It is ideal for anyone eager to build a foundation for good health - now and for the years to come.

Alkaline Diet Plan - A Way to Prevent

Premature Aging

When I reached the age of 25, I always felt sick and weak. I had a hard time to figure out what the causes of my health problems were. I consulted with more than one doctor, yet the illness was still there. The alkaline diet plan has been the best remedy for my health problem.

I have experienced premature aging at the age of 25. I came to know that the main cause of premature aging is too much acidity in our body. If you are always eating more of the acid foods than alkaline foods, your body becomes acidic. There are some symptoms that can be seen during premature aging.

Among These Symptoms Are:

1. Weakness and Fatigue.

Weakness and fatigue are associated with premature aging. Too much acid intake may cause an unhealthy lifestyle. Drinking alcohols and smoking are not good for your health. Alcohols are acid forming drinks. Cigars fall under acid category too.

You will not see the effect of your too much acid intake at an early stage. However, when this stuff began to accumulate in the body, they will cause illness. And these illnesses are shown by symptoms such as weakness and fatigue.

I am not used to drinking and smoking, though I may say, I used to include dairy products in my everyday snacks. I even did not include lots of fruits and vegetables in my previous diet. Stress from work also caused my body system to be more acidic.

2. Aches and pains in the body.

When you feel pain anywhere in your body, it means that something is wrong. Surely, there is an unbalanced fluid pH. If your body pH is not maintained at its optimum, the cells will not function well.

The body cells need nutrients and minerals to enable them to help our body produce enough energy. If the cells are damaged, our tissues and organs will definitely be compromised too. It is because cells make them up. And organs and tissues make up our body.

We experience pains and aches in our joints and muscles. Oftentimes, when we experience premature aging, we suffer from arthritis and other bone diseases. In turn, we cannot do our tasks.

3. Emotional disturbances like depression.

Too much acidity causes emotional disturbance. If you do not eat the right foods, you will not have a healthy body. If you do not have a healthy body, it means that you do not have a healthy mind too. The alkaline diet plan is the answer to having a healthy mind and body. Together with regular exercises, you can achieve a healthy lifestyle. Alkaline foods help your blood to deliver oxygen and other nutrients properly. Exercise also helps oxygen to be delivered uniformly in the body.

Acid foods hinder our blood to carry the oxygen all throughout our body. It is because they let the red blood cells clump together. In effect, it gets harder for them to pass through the bloodstream. And the nutrients and oxygen are not delivered properly.

These are the symptoms of premature aging. An alkaline diet plan would best suit someone who suffers from this. And I know for sure, that like me, many people have been experiencing it. I am glad I have overcome this situation.

So, if you feel any discomfort, like aches and pains, you should try this now. You just have to remember that alkaline food to acid food ratio must be 4:1.

The Acid Alkaline Balanced Diet - What is it?

What is the definition of an acid-alkaline balanced diet? You have probably heard of this nutritious way of eating, which is more commonly described as the alkaline diet. In actuality, "acid-alkaline balanced diet" may truly be the aptest name because the purpose of this approach to eating isn't to go to an extreme of alkalinity, but rather to create a balanced internal pH.

With pH, as with many areas of health, balance is important. For instance, take body temperature. Is body heat a bad thing that you want to minimize?

Or is it a good thing that you want to maximize? The truth, of course, is neither. Either too high or too low a body temperature is a sign that the body is imbalanced.

In the same way, a pH that is either too high or too low is a sign that your body is imbalanced. This imbalance is usually the result of an unsuitable diet. And although it is certainly possible for the body to be either too acidic or too alkaline, overacidity (sometimes referred to as chronic low-grade metabolic acidosis) is far more common than alkalosis. This is because the Western diet is strongly tilted toward acid-producing foods.

But on the bright side, you needn't worry about your body becoming too alkaline, as long as you eat a balanced diet and do not overdo it on alkalizing supplements. A balanced alkaline diet provides balanced amounts of fat, protein, and carbohydrates, in addition to both acid-producing and alkaline-producing foods. Fruits and vegetables are emphasized, along with certain whole grains, legumes, nuts and seeds, and healthy oils.

A dramatic change from crazy fad diets, the acid-alkaline balanced diet is a sound pattern of eating that is similar to the way that healthy peoples have eaten for thousands of years.

The Secrets Behind Curing Your GERD With an Alkaline Diet

Is it really possible to cure your GERD with an alkaline diet? Here's some stuff that your doctor or gastroenterologist probably failed to tell you, or spoke in a soft squeaky voice enough for you not to pay any attention to it.

If you have done careful research on conventional methods vs the natural methods of treating GERD or Acid Reflux, you probably know that what conventional medicine is more after is treating your symptoms and masking the pain. More commonly known as the "band-aid" approach, rarely does it look for the root problem.

People who are suffering from this condition or any digestive disorder for that matter know this. They visit their doctor, receive a consultation, get a series of tests (e.g. ultrasound, blood test, endoscopy - which is normal and highly recommendable), come up with an accurate diagnosis, and then what? You guessed it right. Here come the endless prescriptions, ranging from antacids to purple pills, and liquid stuff that's supposed to keep your acid-locked up where it should be, and out of the esophageal area.

And the cycle repeats itself until either one of two things happens. You are "cured" from your GERD, only to find it re-appearing later in your life and at a far worse condition than when you started treatment. Or the medicines don't work, you rush back to your doctor and what does he do? He gives you a stronger dose of the same medication, and/or adds to that another pill that he claims will do so and so, and aid this and that. Yup, the "band-aid" approach. Never worked for me.

The natural approach, on the other hand, focuses on just what exactly is the problem and addresses it head-on. A alkaline diet is just one of the many tried and proven treatments that are available to cure your GERD because, in reality, it is not a disease but a condition. You can't cure a disease, but you can most definitely cure a condition.

Here are some things that can help you cure your GERD with an alkaline diet -

1. For the first few days, go on a soft liquid diet. This is to allow your esophagus time to rest and heal itself. Avoid eating all spicy and fried foods. Don't worry, this isn't forever. Drink one tablespoon of honey before bedtime, and if experiencing any symptoms of reflux.

2. Make it a habit to avoid all forms of highly acidic foods. There are food charts available that list groups from slightly acidic, to acidic and highly acidic.

. Likewise, do the exact opposite. Go for foods that are highly alkaline. Here's a list of some very alkaline foods to give you a headstart: asparagus, broccoli, grapefruit, lemons, mangoes, onions, parsley, spinach, ginger tea, fresh vegetable juices, watercress, and yellow beans

Practice proper food combining consistently - let's face it. It's hard to eat one type of food group alone. That's what this is for. Proper food combining shows you what types of foods are compatible with each other, and help you experience painless digestion (something that you may have missed already if you have been suffering from acid reflux for a long time).

Digestive disorders such as GERD are the #1 reason people visit their doctors today. The #1 reason.

But are you Curing your Acid Reflux Disease, or making it worse? I hate to admit it, but when I learned what conventional medicine was actually doing to my body, I was enraged!

CHAPTER:-8
ALKALINE DIET CAN SAVE YOUR LIFE

The theory behind the alkaline diet is that because the pH of our body is slightly alkaline, with a normal range of 7.36 to 7.44, our diet should reflect this, and also be slightly alkaline. An unbalanced diet high in acidic foods like animal protein, caffeine, sugar, and processed foods tend to upset this balance. It can deplete the body of alkaline minerals such as sodium, potassium, magnesium, and calcium, making people vulnerable to chronic and degenerative diseases.

Our internal chemical balance is mainly controlled by our lungs, kidneys, intestines, and skin. For necessary functions to occur, our body must maintain a proper pH. The measure of the acidity or alkalinity of a substance is called pH. Adequate alkaline reserves are required for optimal adjustment of pH. The body needs oxygen, water, and acid-buffering minerals to accomplish the pH-buffering while quickly removing waste products.

The over-acidification of the body is the underlying cause of all diseases. Soda is probably the most acidic food people consume at a pH of 2.5. Soda is 50,000 times more acidic than neutral water and takes 32 glasses of neutral water to balance a glass of soda.

Alkaline food and water should be consumed, in order to provide nutrients the body needs to neutralize acids and toxins from the blood, lymph, and tissues, and at the same time, strengthens the immune and organ systems.

Most vegetables and fruits contain a higher amount of alkaline forming elements than other foods. The greater the number of green foods consumed in the diet, the greater the health benefits achieved.

These plant foods are cleansing and alkalizing to the body, while the refined and processed foods can increase unhealthy levels of acidity and toxins.

But be aware that too much alkaline can also harm you. You must have the proper knowledge of balancing alkaline and acidic foods in your diet. After ingestion, alkaline food and water are almost immediately neutralized by hydrochloric acid present in the stomach. The balance between alkaline and acidic foods must be maintained in order for your organs to perform well.

An healthy and balanced diet is more alkaline than acid. Based upon your blood type, the diet should be made up of 60 to 80% alkaline foods and 20 to 40% acidic foods. Normally, the A and AB blood types require the most alkaline diet while the O and B blood types require more animal products in their diet. But keep in mind; if you're in pain, you're acidic.

Transitioning to an alkaline diet requires a shift in one's attitude about food. It is helpful to explore new tastes and textures while making small changes and improving old habits.

CHAPTER:-9
ALKALINE DIET IN GENERAL

The theory explains that upon eating alkaline rich food it leaves an alkaline residue or ash. Now, this ash is considered a mineral containing the principal elements like calcium, iron, magnesium, copper, and zinc these elements contributes to maintaining the homeostasis of the body. Acidifying foods cause these essential minerals to drop in levels predisposing our body to various illnesses engaging to alkaline diet protects the body and prevents that from happening. Basically, our body should maintain a pH of 7.3, meaning to say, our body needs to be alkaline in nature and it should also reflect in our food intake. Alkaline diet doesn't just shed the extra pounds off but over and above that, it regains loss health and promotes long and disease-free life.

Enticing, Exquisite And Flavorful Recipes to Maintain An Alkaline Diet

Alkaline diet recipes include a higher level of vegetable intake, a squeeze of lemon into water drinks, millet or quinoa should replace wheat and olive oil over vegetable oil, soups like miso best follow the diet. Whipping up a savory lunch with a cucumber salad - the ingredients are fresh tomatoes and cucumbers, balsamic vinegar, red wine, sea salt, minced garlic, fresh basil and oregano, and extra virgin olive oil. For dinner, you can make vegetable pasta with tomato-pepper sauce all you need is a vegetable or spelled pasta, sun-dried and fresh tomatoes, red bell pepper, zucchini, onion and garlic, chili, fresh basil, cold-pressed olive oil, and salt and pepper to taste (the vegetables are stir-fried and use it as a topping to the pasta).

Now, a meal would not be complete without a dessert, here are some of the guilt-free desserts that can surely satisfy your cravings like apple pie - you will need ground raw walnuts, pitted dates soaked in alkaline water for 15 minutes, raw sunflower seeds, shredded apples, cinnamon, fresh apple juice, shredded coconut for garnishing, and raisins or prunes. All the dry ingredients, even the ones soaked and drained, should be mixed in a food processor and will serve as the crust. For a quicker dessert you can layer strawberries, blueberries, raspberries, blackberries, plain yogurt, and wheat germ and almonds for garnish a "berry" delightful dessert indeed!

Find out the 3 simple alkalizing steps you can use right now to instantly gain more vibrant health, energy and optimal weight - FAST...

Quick and Easy Alkaline Diet Shortcuts

An alkaline diet can be one of the best ways of increasing your overall health and sense of well-being. Although some people mistakenly think that "eating alkaline" is complicated and difficult to do, it's actually very easy to switch your diet from one that is overly acid to one that is healthy and alkaline. If you want to experience the many health benefits of an alkaline diet, there are some quick and easy ways to get fast results. You can experience better health, better disease resistance, and an increased level of energy, among other benefits, simply from switching to an alkaline diet.

Add Alkaline Water to Your Diet

Drinking plenty of water is essential to good health, so why not make the most of it by drinking alkaline water? It's easy to make your own water at home, simply by adding about a half teaspoon of baking soda to a gallon jug of water.

Shake and test with a pH strip, adding more baking soda if needed to achieve a pH of 8.5 to 9. Or, use alkaline drops, tablets, or a jug filter, which are all commercially available. You can also purchase a water ionizer to attach directly to your water supply for the ultimate in convenience. For a delicious and alkalizing drink, add a squeeze of fresh lemon to your alkaline water before drinking. You can also use it to make healthy herbal and green teas, both of which are alkaline beverages.

Eat Plenty of Salads

Salads made from lettuce, spinach, and other leafy green vegetables are great alkaline diet additions. By simply adding a fresh vegetable salad to your lunch and dinner menu, you'll be improving your health as well as alkalizing your body. Almost all vegetables are alkalizing, so you'll have plenty of choices to keep your salads interesting and exciting. Try adding sliced cucumbers, snow peas, fresh green peas, and green pepper strips to your salad. You can even add a bit of protein by including beans and other legumes.

Eat Less Sugar

Refined sugar is very detrimental to one's health, especially since it encourages an acidic response within the body. If you are accustomed to the sweetness that white sugar provides, try cutting it back gradually so that your taste buds have a chance to adjust. You can also replace white processed sugar with a bit of raw sugar, maple sugar or Stevia, which are all alkalizing sweetening choices. However, don't replace sugar with artificial sweeteners such as Equal, NutraSweet or Sweet 'N Low, since they are acidifying. Fortunately, as you start to cut back on sweeteners, you'll find that you actually start to prefer a less sweet flavor in your foods.

Easy Food Substitutions

It's easy to change your diet from being highly acidifying to alkalizing by just making a few simple food replacements. Instead of processed noodles and pasta, eat whole grains such as millet, quinoa, and wild rice. Replace the red meat in your diet with fish, beans and other legumes for protein. Use healthy fats in your foods, such as olive, flaxseed, or canola oil. You should also eat a diet that is rich in fresh fruits and vegetables since most are alkalizing. Before you know it, you'll be feeling better and reaping the health benefits of an alkaline diet.

Dangers of the Alkaline Diet - What Are They?

Have you heard of the Alkaline diet? Do you know that it is more popular than even the South Beach Diet? This is one of the most trendy diets for losing weight and becoming more healthy. However, are their dangers of the alkaline diet?

The alkaline diet is very effective and it will allow you to return to your ideal weight for your height and body style. This type of diet is made to raise your energy levels and to make you feel better overall.

However, even with the best of diets, there are some risks or dangers involved. So what should you be worried about when it comes to the dangers of the alkaline diet?

The first thing you have to know is that you cannot be on the alkaline diet 100%. You need to have some acidic foods in your body and it is not a bad thing to eat some meat. Most people do not understand that with any diet it is all about balance. You cannot maintain a healthy way of life without some balance.

The next thing you need to know is that this type of diet does not address some of the essential nutrients you need. The alkaline diet does not include fatty acids and things like Omega 3 that you need in your body. This is, again, where the balance comes in. You can have things that are not considered part of the alkaline diet and you just have to balance them out with good alkaline foods and liquids.

The last danger you need to understand is you cannot be poisoning yourself. This is a bit strange to think about, but drinking bottled water or tap water could have certain toxins that are not good for your body. The plastic has chemicals in it and they are not good for your body. The best way to go is to use a filtration system and add a slice of fresh lemon or lime to your water to make is alkaline.

Alkaline Diet Tips - How to Get The Most Out Of It

An alkaline diet involves ensuring that over 80% of the total food intake comprises of alkalizing foods. This diet is easily followed if fruits and vegetables form a major part of one's diet so that illness can be reversed and the aging process slowed down. Even though there are ways to find out what the alkalizing foods are it may still get a bit difficult to incorporate the alkaline diet in our daily regime. If certain tips of an alkaline diet are kept in mind the diet is easy to follow as well as maintain as a part of our lifelong daily schedule.

Water and citrus juices are both alkalizing food. So when on this diet squeeze a lemon in your glass of water as frequently as you can. Lemon though essentially an acidic fruit is alkalizing for the body. It gets cumbersome to make lemonade each time and also sugar is involved (unless one uses stevia). To avoid all pains yet get the gains of the alkaline diet a lemon squeezed in water will take care of both mineral water as well as lemons.

One of the easiest ways to follow an alkaline diet is to eatan lot of fruits and vegetables. Irrespective of what meal one is having one should try and consume an lot of vegetables and fruits. Instead of filling up on bread have a huge bowl of sautéed vegetables or even a large cabbage salad could do wonders for your body's ph level. Thoroughly cleaned fruits are a simple substitute for those nasty and acidic evening snacks. Try having an apple or a peach instead of a packet of chips. It also helps to put one cup of alkalizing greens aside to consume during the day. A cup of broccoli or kale kept aside and eaten during the day will ensure the intake of vegetables.

Wheat is acidic food. When on the alkaline diet substitute millet or quinoa for wheat. White bread should also be discarded as they are acidic foods too. When craving for that lovely meat dish chooses chicken over beef. Have an occasional fish or lamb but try and keep beef off the dining table completely. Just use chicken instead of other meats in the various meat recipes and you shall be good.

Olive oil is very alkalizing and beneficial in ways more than one. When on an alkaline diet discard vegetable and other oils in favors of Olive oil. Use is to get glowing skin and luscious hair too. Consume an lot of greens and add greens powder to almost any dish. Miso is highly alkaline food and a broth can be made simply by adding a teaspoon of it in hot water. This broth can greatly enhance the alkaline levels of the body.

A alkaline diet is easy to follow and can be adopted as an lifestyle rather than a crash diet. It works to keep one's weight in control as well as extend ones life span. A healthy life makes everything worthwhile.

CHAPTER:-10
KNOWING THE DOS AND DON'T
OF THE AKALINE DIET

Most of the diets we know are geared towards weight loss. After all, millions of people around the world are looking for diet tricks to get leaner and look better. The alkaline diet isn't different either, except that it also promotes a 'disease-free' life. Does it work? To know that, it is important to understand that the alkaline diet promotes eating alkaline food. As such, there are a few dos and don'ts in the diet, some of which are extreme, especially if you are someone who lives on meat and dairy. In this post, we will talk about the alkaline diet and some of these dos and don'ts in detail.

The Dos:

The alkaline diet can be called a natural diet because it contains a considerable about of fruits and veggies. So, your diet should essentially consist of fruits and veggies, and most of the available options are allowed. You can also include some of the soy products, including tofu and soybeans. Other things that must be on your list include a few nut varieties, seeds, and some of the lentils and legumes. As for grains, there are a few restrictions, which you can find online. Some experts have promoted the use of vitamin-enhanced water. Basically, this is high pH water that may benefit your body in the same way as these alkaline promoting foods.

The Don'ts:

If you intend to follow the alkaline diet, the don'ts probably matter more than the dos. First things first, cut down meat and dairy from your diet completely. You also need to get off eggs and all sorts of canned, processed and packaged food that you can think of, including your chips, ready meals, and even popcorn. Just check a few books on the alkaline diet, and you will realize that alcohol is not allowed either. You also need to cut down tea and coffee from your diet and all other drinks that may contain caffeine.

Will I Lose Weight?

Now that's a question that most people ask, mainly because this is one of those high-effort diets. The alkaline diet isn't any magic. It doesn't promise rapid weight loss as the GM diet or other similar diets, but since you will be eating more fresh foods, your weight will drop considerably. Also, cutting down processed food makes a significant difference too. With processed and junk food, you are also limiting your sugar intake, which again impacts the weight loss process.

Why The Alkaline Diet? What It Has To Offer You

There has been a lot of talk over the alkaline diet, especially as of late. It seems there is always one diet or another that is the new fad, but this one has long been one of the most popular. For one thing, the point of this diet is not just to achieve rapid loss, but instead to promote healthy living for the long term. This is important because this is not something that can be said for most other diets, whose goal is to help people lose weight as quickly as possible and which are very unhealthy for the body overall.

For the alkaline diet, you need to base your meals around fresh fruits and vegetables. These are the foods that provide the body with the most nutrients, and therefore should be the main components of the diet. This diet has been around longer than almost all other diets. There are a few reasons in particular as to why a person would find this diet helpful. People with a low energy level can feel more energized and awake after sticking to it for a few weeks.

Even different studies have been performed using the alkaline diet to test it and these studies showed it was effective. This is especially true considering that most people live on the altered Western diet which is high in fatty, sugary, processed foods. You want to make sure that you know what you are doing and that you are not cutting out foods that are important to keep your body healthy. People with kidney problems should avoid this diet because it can create problems.

If you are a good candidate for this diet, then you will need to go through your cupboards and start by getting rid of all the bad food. Most people are surprised at just how much unhealthy food they have in their homes. This is also important because it will help keep you from being tempted. You want to get rid of all this temptation and really devote yourself if you want to stick to the alkaline diet.

In terms of results, you will notice them almost immediately when you are on the alkaline diet. The effects are so positive that most people find it easy to stay on the diet after they notice the first sign of any change. Make sure you are exercising regularly along with your alkaline diet for the best results. It certainly offers many benefits over other diets out there today.

CHAPTER:-11
REASONS TO SWITCH TO AN
ALKALINE DIET

E veryone wants to feel good and have their bodies operating at optimal performance, well this is the way to go if you want to look good and feel great! The three reasons that you should switch are fatigue and lack of energy, Inability to lose weight, and finally premature aging (looking and feeling older).

Fatigue and Lack of Energy

Many people are tired and need to find ways to boost their energy level. Switching to an alkaline diet will help with this. Try to eat at least 80% of alkaline foods to the ratio of 20% acid foods and then slowly increase the acid foods to 25-30%. This will boost your energy much more than other more conventional measures.

Inability to Lose Weight

Another reason why people switch to the alkaline diet is that they have an inability to lose weight and they need help. By choosing alkaline foods to eat like vegetables, wheatgrass, and fruit (grapefruit, lemon, lime are good) you will achieve effortless, abundant weight loss.

Other alkaline foods are nuts (almonds), fish oil, coconut oil, flaxseed oil and liver oil, grains like buckwheat, quinoa, and spelling, and condiments like Sea Salts, red chili peppers and most herbs and spices.

Goat's milk, beans and legumes, pumpkin seeds and sesame seeds are also great sources for restoring alkaline balance.

You must also remember to drink plenty of water and take the right supplements to assist your body in balancing your pH.

There is a product out on the market now called Energy Green, it is a supplement. It has many alkaline foods that are part of its ingredients. So there would be no need to consume each item on the list of alkaline foods. But everything is in this one product so this is a plus.

Premature Aging

The more acid you have in your body, the more your body will try to compensate and try to restore its sensitive pH balance by taking the calcium away from your bones, teeth, and tissue. Calcium is only of the 4 alkaline elements that bring the alkaline pH level up in your body and the acid levels down.

There are some experts that think that the reason we age so fast has to do with the number of acidic foods that we eat. Their theory is that we get older because we do not effectively rid our bodies of the wastes and toxins that have accumulated inside our bodies.

The idea is to stop aging and reverse the effects of acidic damage on your body's cells. For this, you should start alkalizing your body according to the acid alkaline diet plan. You must help your body to rid itself of the acid wastes.

So here it is folks, here is hoping that this article has helped many of you dear readers to decide if an alkaline diet is right for you. If you do choose to start this diet, Kudos to you for cleaning up your life and wanting to live healthy for yourself and for your children.

The Theory of the Alkaline Diet

To keep your body fresh and free of diseases, you have to eat the proper food called alkaline diet or acid alkaline diet. Basically, it is a theory that when we eat or consume food, after several processes like digestion, metabolism, and others, it leaves an alkaline residue or acid residue, which determines the acid-alkaline nature of our body.

Alkaline diet theory is based on the fact that the pH of our body is slightly alkaline, that is from 7.35 to 7.45 (in some texts it is 7.36 to 7.44). Our diet should represent this balance. A disturbance in this balance will cause some severe problems in the body. The nature of liquid whether acidic or alkaline is determined by the pH scale. It ranges from 0 (very strong acid) to 14 (very strong alkaline). 7 is the neutral point on pH as that of water. A pH below 7 shows acid things, as we go down, becoming strong acidic, and pH above seven represents alkaline products, the intensity increasing as we go up to 14.

Medical study of almost every kind has alkaline diet roots although this theory not acknowledges by conventional medical societies. Diets which contain 60% alkalinity should be used to maintain the balance of the body. One has to use highly alkaline diets (80%) is the balance of his/her body is disturbed by the extensive use of meat, eggs, cream, and other acidic foods.

Vegetables, low-fat fruits, nuts, tubers fresh citrus and other things should be preferred when talking about alkaline diets. To increase alkalinity in the body, fruits can be used as a good source as most fruits are rich in alkaline. Very few numbers of fruit are acidic. When eating fruits for this purpose, do not eat canned, or sugared or preserved fruits, because they become highly acidic when preserved due to the use of different chemicals.

Vegetables are highly recommended in alkaline diet theory as they are a very good source of making the body alkaline. You will feel weakness rather than power in your body if the meat you are eating to gain energy become an acid forming agent in your body, as conventional doctors do not believe in eating vegetables could be useful and persist on eating meat for energy.

Vegetables, especially green vegetables, are a very good source of alkaline production and you can use them not only cooked, but vegetables like carrot, cauliflower, tomatoes, and others are used any time you want without even cooking. They are tasty and provide you with lots of minerals. Minerals like calcium, potassium, and magnesium are the real source of alkaline ash and are very good for the growth and functioning of the body. Our body is turned from acidic to slightly alkaline when these minerals react with the acid present in our body.

CHAPTER:-12
ALKALINE DIET CHART

T he alkaline acid is a new diet that is gaining more and more popularity. The diet is based upon natural or holistic healing methods and has been around for quite some time. Lately, though, it has been gaining popularity and not just among health nuts. I decided to put together an alkaline diet chart to display what food is considered to be alkaline and healthful and which ones are considered acidic and should be avoided!

Highly Alkaline Foods According to the Alkaline Diet Chart

-Tangerine, Pineapple, Lotus Root, sea salt, lentils, Seaweed, watermelon, tangerine, baking soda, onion, seaweed, mineral water, sweet potato, lime, nectarine, persimmon, raspberry, pumpkin seeds, sea vegetables

Moderately Alkaline Foods according to the Alkaline Diet Chart

-kombucha, broccoli, grapefruit, cantaloupe, citrus, olive, loganberry, parsnip, unsulfured molasses, soy sauce, cashews, grapefruit, cantaloupe, honeydew, garlic, kale, parsley, endive, kohlrabi, chestnuts, pepper, mustard green, ginger, dewberry, arugula, olive

Low Alkaline Forming Foods According to the Alkaline Diet Chart

-Sesame seed, cherry, rutabaga, cauliflower, mu tea, rice syrup, almonds, blackberry, peach, ginseng, collard greens, rice syrup, papaya, cabbage, sour apples, apple cider, mushrooms, avocado, bell pepper, potato, eggplant, sprouts, sake, primrose, bell pepper, apple cider vinegar

Very Low Alkaline Forming Foods According to the Alkaline Diet Chart

-celery, blueberry , raisin, wild rice, ghee, avocado oil, chive, most seeds, cilantro, currant, umeboshi vinegar, coconut oil, olive oil, duck eggs, cucumber, turnip greens, strawberry, flax oil, ghee, flax oil, beet, lettuces, banana, japonica rice, orange, Brussel sprouts, oats, grain coffee

Very Low Acid Forming Foods According to the Alkaline Diet Chart

-Alcohol, chard, plum, farina, elk, lamb, spelt, game mear, wheat, oil, lima beans, teff, kamut, farina, semolina, white rice, cow milk, balsamic vinegar, milk, seitan, pinto beans, tofu, shellfish, mutton, black tea, white rice, vanilla, navy beans, boar, white beans, mollusks, buckwheat, almond oil, safflower, aduki beans, soy cheese, shellfish, aged cheese, tomatoes, red beans, sesame oil, aduki beans, almond oil

Moderately Acid Forming Foods According to the Alkaline Diet Chart

-Coffee, cranberry, pecans, squid, maize, kernel oil, corn, casein, milk protein, lard, oat bran, chicken, green peas, peanuts, pomegranate, soy milk, barley groats, cranberry, nutmeg, pistachios, chestnut oil, garbanzo beans, pork, mussels, rye, legumes, veal.

Highly Acid Forming foods to avoid at all costs!!!

-pudding, fried foods, walnuts, jam, sweeteners, beer, cola, walnuts, hazelnuts, table salt, ice cream, soybean, beef, hops, malt, soft drinks, vinegar, processed cheese, lobster, sugar, barley, cottonseed oil, pheasant.

Why The Alkaline Diet? What It Has To Offer You

There has been a lot of talk over the alkaline diet, especially as of late. It seems there is always one diet or another that is the new fad, but this one has long been one of the most popular. For one thing, the point of this diet is not just to achieve rapid loss, but instead to promote healthy living for the long term. This is important because this is not something that can be said for most other diets, whose goal is to help people lose weight as quickl as possible and which are very unhealthy for the body overall.

For the alkaline diet, you need to base your meals around fresh fruits and vegetables. These are the foods that provide the body with the most nutrients, and therefore should be the main components of the diet. This diet has been around longer than almost all other diets. There are a few reasons in particular as to why a person would find this diet helpful. People with a low energy level can feel more energized and awake after sticking to it for a few weeks.

Even different studies have been performed using the alkaline diet to test it and these studies showed it was effective.

This is especially true considering that most people live on the altered Western diet which is high in fatty, sugary, and processed foods. You want to make sure that you know what you are doing and that you are not cutting out foods that are important to keep your body healthy. People with kidney problems should avoid this diet because it can create problems.

If you are a good candidate for this diet, then you will need to go through your cupboards and start by getting rid of all the bad food. Most people are surprised at just how much unhealthy food they have in their homes. This is also important because it will help keep you from being tempted. You want to get rid of all this temptation and really devote yourself if you want to stick to the alkaline diet.

In terms of results, you will notice them almost immediately when you are on the alkaline diet. The effects are so positive that most people find it easy to stay on the diet after they notice the first sign of any change. Make sure you are exercising regularly along with your alkaline diet for the best results. It certainly offers many benefits over other diets out there today.

CHAPTER:-13
THE ROLE OF PH IN THE BODY

T he pH in our body may vary considerably from one area to another with the highest acidity in the stomach (pH of 1.35 to 3.5) to aid in digestion and protect against opportunistic microbial organisms. But even in the stomach, the layer just outside the epithelium is quite basic to prevent mucosal injury. It has been suggested that decreased gastric lining secretion of bicarbonates and a decrease in the alkaline/acid secretion in duodenal ulcer patients may play a significant role in duodenal ulcers.

The skin is quite acidic (pH 4–6.5) to provide an acid mantle as a protective barrier to the environment against microbial overgrowth. There is a gradient from the outer horny layer (pH 4) to the basal layer (pH 6.9). This is also seen in the vagina where a pH of less than 4.7 protects against microbial overgrowth.

The urine may have a variable pH from acid to alkaline depending on the need for balancing the internal environment. Acid excretion in the urine can be estimated by a formula described by Remer (sulfate + chloride + 1.8x phosphate + organic acids) minus (sodium + potassium + 2x calcium + 2x magnesium) mEq.

Foods can be categorized by the potential renal acid loads (PRALs) see Table 2. Fruits, vegetables, fruit juices, potatoes, and alkali-rich and low phosphorus beverages (red and white wine, mineral soda waters) having a negative acid load. Whereas, grain products, meats, dairy products, fish, and alkali poor and low phosphorus beverages (e.g., pale beers, cocoa) have relatively high acid loads.

Measurement of pH of the urine (reviewed in a recent study with two-morning specimens done over a five-year span) did not predict bone fractures or loss of bone

mineral density. However, this may not be reflective of being on an alkaline or acid diet throughout this time.

Chronic Acidosis and Bone Disease

Calcium in the form of phosphates and carbonates represents a large reservoir of the base in our body. In response to an acid load such as the modern diet, these salts are released into the systemic circulation to bring about pH homeostasis. It has been estimated that the quantity of calcium lost in the urine with the modern diet over time could be as high as almost 480 gm over 20 years or almost half the skeletal mass of calcium. However, urinary losses of calcium are not a direct measure of osteoporosis.

There are many regulatory factors that may compensate for the urinary calcium loss. When the arterial pH is in the normal range, a mild reduction of plasma bicarbonate results in a negative calcium balance which could benefit from supplementing bicarbonate in the form of potassium bicarbonate.

It has been found that bicarbonate, which increases the alkali content of a diet, but not potassium may attenuate bone loss in healthy older adults. The bone minerals that are wasted in the urine may not have complete compensation through intestinal absorption, which is thought to result in osteoporosis

However, adequate vitamin D with a 25(OH)D level of >80 nmol/L may allow for appropriate intestinal absorption of calcium and magnesium and phosphate when needed. Sadly, most populations are generally deficient in vitamin D especially in northern climates. In chronic renal failure, correction of metabolic acidosis with bicarbonate significantly improves parathyroid levels and levels of the active form of vitamin D 1,25(OH)2D3.

Recently, a study has shown the importance of phosphate in Remer's PRAL formula. According to the formula, it would be expected that an increase in phosphate should result in an increase in urinary calcium loss and a negative calcium balance in bone. It should be noted that supplementation with phosphate in patients with bed rest reduced urinary calcium excretion but did not prevent bone loss.

The most recent systematic review and meta-analysis have shown that calcium balance is maintained and improved with phosphate which is quite contrary to the acid-ash hypothesis. As well a recent study looking at soda intake (which has a significant amount of phosphate) and osteoporosis in postmenopausal American first nations women did not find a correlation. It is quite possible that the high acid content according to Remer's classification needs to be looked at again in light of compensatory phosphate intake.

There is online information promoting an alkaline diet for bone health as well as a number of books. However, a recent systematic review of the literature looking for evidence supporting the alkaline diet for bone health found no protective role of dietary acid load in osteoporosis.

Another element of the modern diet is the excess of sodium in the diet. There is evidence that in healthy humans the increased sodium in the diet can predict the degree of hyperchloremic metabolic acidosis when consuming a net acid-producing diet. As well, there is evidence that there are adverse effects of sodium chloride in the aging population.

A high sodium diet will exacerbate disuse-induced bone and muscle loss during immobilization by increasing bone resorption and protein wasting. Excess dietary sodium has been shown to result in hypertension and osteoporosis in women. As well, dietary potassium which is lacking in the modern diet would modulate pressor and hypercalciuric effects of excess of sodium chloride.

Excess dietary protein with high acid renal load may decrease bone density if not buffered by ingestion of supplements or foods that are alkali-rich. However, adequate protein is necessary for the prevention of osteoporosis and sarcopenia; therefore, increasing the amount of fruit and vegetables may be necessary rather than reducing protein.

Alkaline Diets and Muscle

As we age, there is a loss of muscle mass, which may predispose to falls and fractures. A three-year study looking at a diet rich in potassium, such as fruits and vegetables, as well as a reduced acid load, resulted in the preservation of muscle mass in older men and women. Conditions such as chronic renal failure that result in chronic metabolic acidosis result in an accelerated breakdown in skeletal muscle.

"Correction of acidosis may preserve muscle mass in conditions where muscle wasting is common such as diabetic ketosis, trauma, sepsis, chronic obstructive lung disease, and renal failure. In situations that result in acute acidosis, supplementing younger patients with sodium bicarbonate prior to exhaustive exercise resulted in significantly less acidosis in the blood than those that were not supplemented with sodium bicarbonate."

Alkaline Supplementation and Growth Horone

It has long been known that severe forms of metabolic acidosis in children, such as renal tubular acidosis, are associated with low levels of growth hormone with resultant short stature. Correction of the acidosis with bicarbonate or potassium citrate increases growth hormone significantly and improved growth.

The use of enough potassium bicarbonate in the diet to neutralize the daily net acid load in postmenopausal women resulted in a significant increase in growth hormone and resultant osteocalcin. Improving growth hormone levels may improve quality of life, reduce cardiovascular risk factors, improve body composition, and even improve memory and cognition. As well this results in a reduction of urinary calcium loss equivalent to 5% of bone calcium content over a period of 3 years.

Alkaline Diet and Back Pain

There is some evidence that chronic low back pain improves with the supplementation of alkaline minerals. With supplementation, there was a slight but significant increase in blood pH and intracellular magnesium. Ensuring that there is enough intracellular magnesium allows for the proper function of enzyme systems and also allows for activation of vitamin D. This, in turn, has been shown to improve back pain.

Alkalinity and Chemotherapy

The effectiveness of chemotherapeutic agents is markedly influenced by pH. Numerous agents such as epirubicin and adriamycin require alkaline media to be more effective. Others, such as cisplatin, mitomycin C, and thiotepa, are more cytotoxic in an acid media. Cell death correlates with acidosis and intracellular pH shifts higher (more alkaline) after chemotherapy may reflect a response to chemotherapy.

It has been suggested that inducing metabolic alkalosis may be useful in enhancing some treatment regimes by using sodium bicarbonate, carbicab, and furosemide. Extracellular alkalinization by using bicarbonate may result in improvements in therapeutic effectiveness . There is no scientific literature establishing the benefit of an alkaline diet for the prevention of cancer at this time.

The human body has an amazing ability to maintain a steady pH in the blood with the main compensatory mechanisms being renal and respiratory. Many of the membranes in our body require an acid pH to protect us and to help us digest food.

It has been suggested that an alkaline diet may prevent a number of diseases and result in significant health benefits. Looking at the above discussion on bone health alone, certain aspects have doubtful benefit.

There does not seem to be enough evidence that milk or cheese may be as detrimental as Remer's formula suggests since phosphate does benefit bone health and result in a positive calcium balance. However, another mechanism for the alkaline diet to benefit bone health may be the increase in growth hormone and the resultant increase in osteocalcin.

There is some evidence that the K/Na ratio does matter and that the significant amount of salt in our diet is detrimental. Even some governments are demanding that the food industry reduce the salt load in our diet.

High-protein diets may also affect bone health but some protein is also needed for good bone health. Muscle wasting, however, seems to be reduced with an alkaline diet and back pain may benefit from this as well. An alkaline environment may improve the efficacy of some chemotherapy agents but not others.

CHAPTER:-14
DAYS ALKALINE DIET PLAN TO HEALTHY WEIGHT LOSS

F irst or second thoughts to go alkaline? It has been years now since I have been advising all my clients to include more and more of Alkaline foods in their diet. If you, perhaps, have caught on to this notion that going alkaline means cutting down other foods completely out of your diet, then you have been misled. Actually, let's not even focus on elimination. Rather, I want to make you ponder about all the appetizing, fresh and nourishing alkaline foods you can eat to boost your overall immunity and health. To show you how I have compiled a seven-day meal plan with world-famous alkaline recipes that use ingredients you already work with all the time

So, according to the science behind this diet, eating specific foods that make your body more alkaline can protect against those conditions as well as shed pounds. Your alkaline diet will include fruits rich in citric acid, all greens, nuts, multigrain (especially oats).

7-day alkaline plant based diet meal plan

- *Monday Meals*
- *Tuesday Tucks*
- *Wednesday Commons*
- *Thursday Greens*
- *Friday Feeds*
- *Saturday Solids*
- *Sunday Scoff*

VEGAN HIGH ALKALINE DIET

1.Why akaline diet is considered good for your body?

Considering having the high alkaline diet is possibly the best decision you could ever make. As you know that the pH level of your body is a fusion of alkalinity or acidity which plays a significant role in your health because overly alkaline or overly acidic conditions can stop your enzymes from working properly. The high alkaline food items affect the pH level of your body and proponents claim focusing on alkaline-forming foods for at least 70% of your daily diet will combat disease and benefit your health. Although there is not enough scientific evidence which exists to back up the health claims which are associated with an alkaline diet I have been personally experiencing its benefits.

Fun Fact: Do you know that the alkaline diet has been into the news since Victoria Beckham tweeted about an alkaline diet cookbook in January 2013?

2. Benefits of an Alkaline Diet Plan

Not all the benefits of the alkaline diet are backed by science. For example, there is no captivating evidence which shows that this alkaline diet can prevent cancer - a common proclaimed health benefit. However, following an alkaline diet can increase the ratio of potassium to sodium in your body, which promotes bone and muscle health, and might also lower your risk of heart disease, the review explains. The typical alkaline diet is also high in magnesium, a mineral essential for cell function. Magnesium also helps your body use vitamin D -- a hormone essential for healthy bones -- so following an alkaline diet might help your body better use vitamin D. An alkaline diet might also increase your levels of growth hormone, a compound important for heart health, as well as cognitive function.

3. Alkaline Foods to Emphasize

At least 70 percent of your diet should come from alkaline-forming foods. This includes almost all vegetables -- with the exception of pickled veggies and sauerkraut. Focus on leafy greens for your alkaline diets, such as wheat grass, sprouts, kale, dandelion, and barley grass. Eat alkaline root veggies, like beetroot, kohlrabi, and radishes. Several fruits are also alkaline-forming, with lime, lemon, avocado, cherries, watermelon and ripe bananas among your best options.

Opt for whole grains like Kamut, buckwheat, millet and spelled, and get alkaline-friendly carbs and protein with lentils. Hydrate with water, as well as herbal and green teas, sweetened with an alkaline sweetener like stevia if needed.

4. Why you should avoid acidic food?

Up to 30 percent of your daily food intake can come from acid-forming foods if you're following an alkaline diet. Limit refined grains such as white bread, and opt instead for whole-grain versions. While whole-wheat bread is still slightly acidic, it's a less acidic option than white bread, corn tortillas or sourdough bread. Eat acidic fruits -- a group that includes mandarins, pineapple, tangerine, raspberries and unripe bananas -- in moderation.

Avoid cooking with acid-forming oils, including butter, margarine, corn oil, and sunflower oil, and steer clear of acid-forming nuts like peanuts and pistachios. Minimize your use of certain condiments, including ketchup, mustard, mayo and soy sauce.

7-day alkaline plant based diet meal plan

Alkaline foods are important so as to bring about a balance. Like all experts and doctors have been saying for years, we should have a balanced meal with a good mix of everything, rather than restraining ourselves to have only a certain category of food items.

You should start your day with a warm glass of water with some lemon juice which will help your body to eliminate toxins. Also, all the ingredients which you will use should be organic to prevent ingesting additional toxins (pesticides/herbicides/GMO laden foods).

Day 1: Monday Meals

Breakfast: Power Smoothie with Chia Porridge

Power Smoothie: Blend the mixture of 2 cups spinach or greens of your choice, 2 cups water or nut milk, 2-4 tablespoons of any Protein powder, ½ tsp of cinnamon which is great for lowering blood sugar, 1 tablespoon of green powder of your choice, of tocotrienols which has a calming effect, colostrum powder (optional) and 1 apple (optional to sweeten). Also, you can soak a ½ cup of chia seeds but you can add it later.

Chia Porridge: Mix chia seeds with warm or cold almond milk, let sit for 2-3 minutes until chia starts to absorb almond milk. Add a splash of vanilla and cinnamon.

Lunch:

Mixed Greens Salad with Red Bell Pepper Dressing and Quinoa

Mixed Greens Salad: Mixed Greens of your choice, 1 large tomato, 1 carrot shredded, 1 cucumber chopped, 1 cup of red bell pepper chopped, 1 avocado, 1 beet shredded (veggies are optional) and add pumpkin seeds, sunflower seeds, etc.

Red Bell Pepper Dressing: Make a big batch and store of 1.5 c chopped red bell pepper, ¼ c carrot, chopped, 1.5 TBS ginger, 1 garlic clove, 1.5

TBS lemon or lime juice, 2.5 TBS apple cider vinegar, 1.5 tsp Himalayan or sea salt, ½ c olive oil, water if needed. Place all ingredients in a blender and store it in a glass jar. Serve over salad, veggie pasta, cooked quinoa or beans for variations you can add Mexican seasoning, Thai flavors, cayenne pepper or Indian spices to complement the meal.

Quinoa: Add quinoa to boiling water, let boil, reduce heat and simmer without a lid for about 20 minutes or until tender. Add more water if quinoa is not fully cooked, but water has dried up. Add Italian seasoning and Himalayan salt (optional) to taste. Can be served as a side or mixed with Green Salad.

Dinner: Pasta Primavera

On a baking sheet toss all veggies (of your choice) with olive oil, sea salt, pepper, dried Italian herbs. Bake about 20 minutes until veggies begin to turn brown. You can also sauté' your veggies. When done, toss with uncooked spiralized zucchini noodles, cooked spelled pasta, or baked spaghetti squash (halved lengthwise and seeded). Put Spaghetti Squash facing down on a baking sheet, bake on 350 degrees for 30 minutes. Scoop spaghetti squash out and toss with veggies. Add fresh basil and chopped cherry tomatoes for taste.

Day 2: Tuesday Tucks

Breakfast: Quinoa with Almond milk and Avocado on Toast

Quinoa with Almond milk: Heat saucepan on medium heat and pour in quinoa, season with cinnamon and cook until quinoa is toasted (2-3 minutes). Stir frequently to avoid burning quinoa.

Add almond milk, water, and vanilla. Bring to a boil then let simmer until the porridge thickens and quinoa is tender (about 25 minutes). If the liquid dries before quinoa is tender, add a little more water. Stir occasionally until done so porridge does not burn.

Avocado on Toast: Take 1 ripe avocado, 1 tsp organic extra virgin olive oil, the juice from ½ lemon, 1 slice of toast (Coconut Bread) and Pepper to taste.

Lunch: Sweet and Savory Salad

Take 1 large head of butter lettuce, ½ cucumber, sliced, 1 pomegranate, seeded or 1/3 cup seeds, 1 avocado, a ¼ cup of chopped shelled pistachios with ¼ cup apple cider vinegar, ½ cup extra virgin olive oil, 1 minced garlic clove. Hand tears the butter lettuce into a salad bowl. Add the rest of the ingredients and toss with the salad dressing.

Dinner: Raw Vegan Pad Thai

Blend all ingredients(raw almond butter, orange juice, fresh ginger, organic coconut aminos or Bragg's Liquid Aminos, in a blender, except Kelp Noodles, until smooth. Drain and rinse Kelp Noodles. Toss with the sauce, add garnishes and a splash of lime juice (not too much). Let your bowl sit for 10 minutes to let Kelp Noodles absorb flavors.

Day 3: Wednesday Commons

Breakfast: Non-Dairy Apple Parfait

Combine cashews, almond milk, and vanilla in a blender and blend until smooth. Layer ingredients in a small cup: a heaping spoon of cashew cream, a spoonful of apples, top with oats and hemp seeds and enjoy!

Lunch: Savory Avocado Wrap

Spread avocado onto the leaf and sprinkle with basil, cilantro, red onion, tomato, salt, and pepper and add spinach. Fold in half and enjoy!

Dinner: Mock Tuna Salad

Place Sunflower seeds in a bowl and cover with cold water, put in refrigerator overnight. Rinse and drain seeds. Put in a food processor with olive oil and sea salt or Himalayan salt, pulse until chunky paste forms. Move mixture to a bowl and stir in remaining ingredients. Serve over a green salad or put in Romaine Lettuce Wrap.

Day 4: Thursday Greens

Breakfast: Almond Butter Crunch Berry Smoothie

Blend spinach and almond milk first. Then add remaining ingredients except for chia, and blend. Add chia once all is smooth – then blend on a very low speed to mix. If you don't have a variable speed blender, mix chia in with the rest of the ingredients by hand. Let sit for a few minutes for the chia seeds to expand, then enjoy.

Lunch: Kale Pesto Pasta

The night before, soak walnuts to improve absorption. Put all ingredients (1 bunch kale, 2 cups fresh basil, 1/4 cup extra virgin olive oil, 1/2 cup walnuts, 2 limes, salt, and pepper) in a blender or food processor, and blend until you get a creamy consistency. Garnish with sliced asparagus, spinach leaves, and tomato (optional). Add to zucchini noodles and enjoy!

Dinner: Butternut Squash Risotto

Preheat Oven 350 degrees and place diced squash on a baking sheet, drizzle with 2 TBS olive oil and bake 15 minutes until creamy. Heat remaining oil in a wide bottomed pan over medium heat. Add onions and garlic, cook stirring constantly for 1 minute to coat the rice in oil. Reduce heat and stir in 2 large ladles of veggie stock. Simmer, stirring gently over low heat until the rice has absorbed the stock.

Continue adding veggie stock one ladle at a time stirring gently until absorbed. Repeat. After 30 minutes, stir in butternut squash & chopped sage leaves. Continue to add veggie stock until the rice is cooked, stirring slowly (about 50 minutes). Serve warm!

Day 5: Friday Feeds

Breakfast: Apple and Almond Butter Oats

Add the oats, coconut milk, and almond butter into a bowl and mix well. Stir in the grated apple; cover the bowl with a lid or plastic wrap and place in the refrigerator. Refrigerate overnight. If the oats get too thick, add some coconut milk to them. Garnish with cinnamon powder.

Lunch: Green Goddess Bowl with Avocado Cumin Dressing

Lightly steam kale and broccoli (flash steam for 4 minutes), set aside. Mix zucchini noodles and kelp noodles and toss with a generous serving of smoked avocado cumin dressing. Add cherry tomatoes and toss again. Plate the steamed kale and broccoli and drizzle them with lemon tahini dressing. Top kale and broccoli with the dressed noodles and tomatoes and sprinkle the whole dish with hemp seeds.

Dinner: Layered Veggie Bake

Preheat oven to 340 degrees and place lentils in a small pan, cover with water and bring to a boil then simmer 10-15 minutes until Al Dente (not too mushy). Drain-set aside. Heat olive oil in a large pan. Squash the tomato into the oil to make a tomato base for the sauce(use fork or large spoon). Add garlic, beets, tamari, chives and a pinch of cumin. Add the water and cook over medium heat for 15 minutes or until reduced to a thick sauce.

Add lentils to the pan with a splash more water & simmer for 5 minutes. Layer half the butternut squash & 1/3 of the zucchini in an ovenproof dish. Spread half the lentil sauce over layers of zucchini and squash. Repeat the layers finishing with the remaining zucchini. Brush Zucchini with olive oil then bake for 45 minutes or until veggies are tender.

Day 6: Saturday Solids

Breakfast: Berry Good Spinach Power Smoothie

Blend spinach and almond milk first, then add remaining ingredients (2 cups fresh spinach, 2 cups unsweetened almond milk, 1 cup frozen mixed berries, 1 frozen banana, 1 tbsp. coconut oil, ½ tsp. cinnamon, 2 tbsp. raw almond butter and blend.

Lunch: Quinoa Burrito Bowl, FAVORITE!)

Cook quinoa or rice. While cooking, warm beans over low heat. Stir in onions, lime juice, garlic, and cumin and let flavors combine for 10-15 minutes. When quinoa is done the cooking, divide into individual serving bowls. Top with beans, avocado, and cilantro.

Dinner: Vegan Cauliflower Pizza Crust

Preheat the oven to 400F and line a baking sheet with parchment paper. Place the cauliflower florets in the bowl of a large food processor fitted with an "S" blade, and pulse until a rice-like texture is created. Pour the cauliflower "rice" into a large sauce pot, add enough water to cover, and bring to a boil. Cover, reduce the heat and allow to cook for 5 minutes.

Drain the liquid, then transfer the cooked cauliflower rice in a freezer-safe bowl.

Place in the freezer to cool for 10 minutes. In the meantime, mix together 2 tablespoons of ground chia or flax seeds with 6 tablespoons of water, to create a vegan "egg." Set aside and allow the mixture to thicken. Remove the cooled cauliflower rice from the freezer and transfer it to the center of a thin dish towel.

Use your hands to squeeze the rice in the dish towel, removing all of the excess moisture from the cauliflower.

Day 7: Sunday Scoffs

Breakfast: Breakfast Burrito

Add the vegan butter to a hot sauté pan. Sauté' the onions, mushrooms, and pepper for a few minutes. Add in the tempeh and remaining ingredients (all except the spinach and Daiya cheese). Sauté the tempeh and veggies for about 5 minutes - chopping the tempeh adding Himalayan salt and pepper to taste. When tempeh has reached the consistency you like, fold in the spinach to wilt. Turn off heat.

Then fold in the Daiya cheese. It will melt against hot tempeh. Warm your wrap in the pan. Add your scramble to your warmed wrap and fold. You can add extra cheese if you'd like. Serve warm. Salsa or hot sauce on the side is nice.

Lunch: Asian Sesame Dressing and Noodles

In a mixing bowl, combine all the dressing ingredients and thoroughly mix with a spoon. Make your zucchini noodles with a spiralizer or, if using kelp noodles, place in warm water for 10 minutes to rinse off the liquid they are packaged with, allowing them to separate and soften. Add the

Asian Sesame dressing to the noodles and scallions, and mix thoroughly. Add sesame seeds on top, and serve.

Dinner: Detox Lime-Chili Stir 'Fry'

Pulp the coriander with a pestle and mortar along with the finely chopped chili, adding lime juice as you go to make a dressing/sauce. Then set aside to infuse. Now chop all of the vegetables fairly finely (so that they will cook quickly). Steam these until they are only just cooked (still a little crunchy). Now place all ingredients on a bed of fluffy, steamed rice and cover with the coriander and lime-chili sauce.

While concluding the article, I would like to ask you what extra efforts you have done to shed your extra weight? Have they worked out for you? No, right? Because people generally focus on 'what NOT to eat' rather than focusing on 'what to eat'. It is not a healthier way to shed your weight and definitely not a happy one.

I hope the information provided above will work as your personal guide book and will lead you towards the direction of healthy weight loss. It's time for you to follow something which you could tailor into your lifestyle. Because let's be real skipping meals and spending time in the gym won't help unless you switch to an alkaline diet.

CHAPTER:-15
WHAT YOU SHOULD KNOW
ABOUT ALKALINE DIET

W hat You Should Know About the Alkaline Diet Before You Try It

The alkaline diet's premise is this: Replace acidic foods with alkaline foods and your health will improve. Why would that work, you ask? The theory is that by controlling your body's pH level (pH is a scientific scale on which acids and bases are measured), you can lose weight and avoid chronic diseases like cancer and heart disease. Also a consideration in some skin care routines, pH levels are measured on a scale from 1 to 14; under seven are the more acidic foods like vinegar, animal fats, and dairy. Over seven are alkaline foods—these mostly include healthful, plant-based foods. When you digest food, the leftover residue is ash, which can be acidic or alkaline. This is why the alkaline diet is sometimes called the alkaline ash diet. According to proponents of the alkaline diet, acidic ash can be dangerous to your health.

Can changing my diet affect my pH levels?

Yes and no. Many experts are quick to point out that you can't change the pH in your blood by what you eat. "The body is very well tuned to keep the proper pH level throughout—more acidic in the stomach, more neutral or alkaline in the blood—but the body does this on its own and no evidence indicates that diet has much impact, other than short-term during digestion," says Connie Diekman MEd, RD, LD, FADA, director of University Nutrition at Washington University in St. Louis past president of the American Dietetic Association (now the Academy of Nutrition and

Dietetics). You can change the pH of your urine, but urine pH fluctuates quickly and easily and is influenced by many factors other than diet. It is also possible to change the pH level of your saliva by what you eat.

Is the alkaline diet healthy?

Processed meats rank high on the list of foods cancer doctors never eat and are also frowned upon in an alkaline diet because of their high acidity. "An alkaline diet is one that tries to balance the pH level of the body by increasing consumption of alkalizing foods, such as fruits and veggies, and reducing/eliminating most acidic foods, such as processed meats and refined grains," explains says Josh Axe, DNM, author of Eat Dirt and co-founder of Ancient Nutrition. These are the best and worst days to start a diet, according to science.

Will I lose weight on an alkaline diet?

Yes, but it's not magic, says Diekman. "An alkaline diet can lead to weight loss since it limits many higher calorie foods and focuses on lots of fruits and vegetables," she says. There's a catch. "The problem is that it is extreme in what you must avoid making it hard to follow the diet in the real world and it can lead to nutrient gaps due to the elimination of foods that it classifies as too acidic." If you are trying to lose weight, these tiny diet changes can help.

Is an alkaline diet good for teeth?

Smile-friendly alkaline foods raise the pH level in your mouth via saliva and may improve your oral health as a result. Smile-challenging foods are acidic can erode your teeth. Live with acid reflux? If so, this may also affect the health of your smile. That's the main message of a study in General Dentistry, which linked acid reflux to the erosion of tooth enamel. See a dentist if you are concerned.

Can an alkaline diet improve bone health?

Many alkaline diet state that consuming a lot of acid-forming foods can causes calcium to be leached out of bones to maintain the body's pH balance. This is true-ish, experts say. Calcium is a base, which neutralizes acidity. The more acid you consume or make, the more calcium (base) you need to neutralize it, but many other factors play a role in how and when calcium is released from bones. There is no hard-and-fast evidence that an alkaline diet protects the bones, but certain foods and beverages that are restricted on this diet do in fact decrease calcium absorption and lead to bone loss, namely caffeine and alcohol, according to the National Osteoporosis Foundation.

Can an alkaline diet improve heart health?

There are many habits that can make for a heart-healthy day, and eating a diet that is largely plant-based (like the alkaline diet) is known to be good for the heart. The alkaline diet is also low in animal protein and processed meats which are loaded with sodium and can increase blood pressure in some people. The alkaline also eliminates such waistline saboteurs as processed foods and sweets. High blood pressure and obesity are major risk factors for heart disease. These are the best and worst diets for heart health.

Can an alkaline diet lower cancer risk?

Many cancer-fighting foods are also alkaline diet foods, but at this point, there is no evidence for or against the role that an alkaline diet can play in cancer prevention. A plant-based diet, however, is believed to help lower risk for cancer and is even recommended for cancer survivors, according to the American Cancer Research Institute.

New research out the University of Alabama at Birmingham shows that a plant-based diet may make it easier to treat one of the more the most lethal breast cancers. Though the evidence is a bit conflicting: Certain chemotherapy drugs kill more cancer cells in an alkaline environment and others work better in an acidic one, according to a review study in the Journal of Environmental Public Health. This is something to discuss with your doctor if you are being treated for cancer.

Will an alkaline diet improve back pain?

here are many surprising causes of back pain, and an acid-rich diet may be one of them. In fact, a study of 82 people with chronic low back pain showed that those who took an alkaline supplement that contained magnesium had less pain than their counterparts who didn't. This alkaline mineral neutralizes the acid and helps muscles relax and may relieve pain as a result. Learn about the best diet for every decade of life.

Getting started on an alkaline diet plan

Add at least some fresh fruits and veggies to all your meals and snacks, Axe says. Try a "meatless Monday" as you aim for more plant-based protein and less meat, especially processed meats. Lower your intake of sodium from processed, canned or frozen foods. Add pH drops, fresh lemon or lime juice, or even baking soda to your water in order to boost its alkalinity. "Don't over-consume alcohol or caffeine by sticking to one alcoholic or caffeinated drink per day or less," he says.

CONCLUSION

Alkaline diets result in a more alkaline urine pH and may result in reduced calcium in the urine, however, as seen in some recent reports, this may not reflect total calcium balance because of other buffers such as phosphate. There is no substantial evidence that this improves bone health or protects from osteoporosis. However, alkaline diets may result in a number of health benefits as outlined below

Increased fruits and vegetables in an alkaline diet would improve the K/Na ratio and may benefit bone health, reduce muscle wasting, as well as mitigate other chronic diseases such as hypertension and strokes.

The resultant increase in growth hormone with an alkaline diet may improve many outcomes from cardiovascular health to memory and cognition.

An increase in intracellular magnesium, which is required for the function of many enzyme systems, is another added benefit of the alkaline diet. Available magnesium, which is required to activate vitamin D, would result in numerous added benefits in the vitamin D apocrine/exocrine systems.

Alkalinity may result in added benefit for some chemotherapeutic agents that require a higher pH.

From the evidence outlined above, it would be prudent to consider an alkaline diet to reduce morbidity and mortality of chronic disease that is plaguing our aging population.

One of the first considerations in an alkaline diet, which includes more fruits and vegetables, is to know what type of soil they were grown in since this may significantly influence the mineral content. At this time, there are limited scientific studies in this area, and many more studies are indicated in regards to muscle effects, growth hormone, and interaction with vitamin D.

It is true that many people who have switched to an alkaline diet see significant health improvements. However, do bear in mind that other reasons may be at work:

Most of us do not eat enough vegetables and fruits. According to the Center for Disease and Prevention, only 9% of Americans eat enough vegetables and 13% enough fruits. If you switch to an alkaline diet, you are automatically eating more vegetables and fruits.

After all, they are very rich in phytochemicals, antioxidants, and fiber which are essential to good health. When you eat more vegetables and fruits, you are probably eating less processed foods too.

Eating less dairy and eggs will benefit those who are lactose-intolerant or have a food sensitivity to eggs, which is rather common among the general population.

Eating fewer grains will benefit those who are gluten-sensitive or have leaky gut or an autoimmune disease.

Made in the USA
Middletown, DE
01 May 2022

65092807R00057